Frozen Section Library:
Genitourinary Tract

Frozen Section Library: Genitourinary Tract

Luan D. Truong, MD

The Methodist Hospital and Baylor College of Medicine,
Houston, TX, USA
Weill Medical College of Cornell University,
New York, NY, USA

Steven S. Shen, MD, PhD

The Methodist Hospital, Houston, TX, USA
Weill Medical College of Cornell University,
New York, NY, USA

Jae Y. Ro, MD, PhD

The Methodist Hospital, Houston, TX, USA
Weill Medical College of Cornell University,
New York, NY, USA

Luan D. Truong
Weill Medical College of
    Cornell University
New York, New York, USA
Baylor College of Medicine
    Houston, Texas, USA
The Methodist Hospital
    Houston, Texas, USA

Jae Y. Ro
Weill Medical College of
    Cornell University
New York, New York, USA
The Methodist Hospital
    Houston, Texas, USA

Steven S. Shen
Weill Medical College of
    Cornell University
New York, New York, USA
The Methodist Hospital
    Houston, Texas, USA

Series editor
Philip T. Cagle, MD
Pathology and Laboratory
    Medicine
Weill Medical College of
    Cornell University
New York, New York, USA
The Methodist Hospital
    Houston, Texas, USA

ISBN 978-1-4419-0690-8   ISBN 978-1-4419-0691-5 (eBook)
DOI 10.1007/978-1-4419-0691-5
Springer Dordrecht Heidelberg London New York

Library of Congress Control Number: 2009927724

Printed on acid-free paper

Springer is part of Springer Science+Business Media (www.springer.com)

Series Preface

For over 100 years, the frozen section has been utilized as a tool for the rapid diagnosis of specimens while a patient is undergoing surgery, usually under general anesthesia, as a basis for making immediate treatment decisions. Frozen section diagnosis is often a challenge for the pathologist who must render a diagnosis that has crucial import for the patient in a minimal amount of time. In addition to the need for rapid recall of differential diagnoses, there are many pitfalls and artifacts that add to the risk of frozen section diagnosis that are not present with permanent sections of fully processed tissues that can be examined in a more leisurely fashion. Despite the century-long utilization of frozen sections, most standard pathology textbooks, both general and subspecialty, largely ignore the topic of frozen sections. Few textbooks have ever focused exclusively on frozen section diagnosis and those textbooks that have done so are now out-of-date and have limited illustrations.

The Frozen Section Library series is meant to provide convenient, user-friendly handbooks for each organ system to expedite use in the rushed frozen section situation. These books are small and lightweight, copiously color-illustrated with images of actual frozen sections, highlighting pitfalls, artifacts, and differential diagnosis. The advantages of a series of organ-specific handbooks, in addition to the ease-of-use and manageable size, are that (1) a series allows more comprehensive coverage of more diagnoses, both common and rare, than a single volume that tries to highlight a limited number of diagnoses for each organ and (2) a series allows more detailed insight by permitting experienced authorities to emphasize the peculiarities of frozen section for each organ system.

As a handbook for practicing pathologists, these books will be indispensable aids to diagnosis and avoiding dangers in one of the most challenging situations that pathologists encounter. Rapid consideration of differential diagnoses and how to avoid traps caused by frozen section artifacts are emphasized in these handbooks. A series of concise, easy-to-use, well-illustrated handbooks alleviates the often frustrating and time-consuming, sometimes futile, process of searching through bulky textbooks that are unlikely to illustrate or discuss pathologic diagnoses from the perspective of frozen sections in the first place. Tables and charts will provide guidance for differential diagnosis of various histologic patterns. Touch preparations, which are used for some organs such as central nervous system or thyroid more often than others, are appropriately emphasized and illustrated according to the need for each specific organ.

This series is meant to benefit practicing surgical pathologists, both community and academic, and to pathology residents and fellows; and also to provide valuable perspectives to surgeons, surgery residents, and fellows who must rely on frozen section diagnosis by their pathologists. Most of all, we hope that this series contributes to the improved care of patients who rely on the frozen section to help guide their treatment.

Philip T. Cagle, MD
Series Editor

Preface

Intraoperative pathology consultation remains one of the most challenging and demanding areas in the practice of diagnostic pathology. The need for making an accurate diagnosis under the constraint of time limitation, suboptimal tissue preparation, and incomplete clinical information, is a well -recognized problem. Yet the literature in this area is limited and the practice of intraoperative pathology consultation is thus influenced by variable factors including personal preference, training background, and institutional tradition for both surgeons and pathologists.

This monograph, *Frozen Section Library: Genitourinary Tract*, is a volume in the *Frozen Section Library Series*. Its content reflects personal experience supplemented by the available pertinent literature. It aims at providing a practical and succinct but comprehensive guideline for for the handling of the genitourinary tract specimens including the kidney, ureter, urethra, penis, bladder, prostate, and testis submitted for intraoperative pathology consultation and the interpretation of the morphologic findings. Whenever possible, morphologic "pearls" or clinical vignettes, which may facilitate a correct diagnosis and at the same time help avoid interpretational pitfalls, are provided. The clinical context of the intraoperative pathology consultation, including its reasons, clinical information necessary for interpretation, different surgical techniques pertinent to the submitted tissue specimens, and the expectations from the consulting surgeons, are also emphasized. These considerations should facilitate effective intraoperative communication with the surgical team.

The monograph includes five chapters (kidney, bladder, penis, prostate, and testis). Each chapter first lists the most common reasons for intraoperative pathology consultation, followed by discussion on the clinical setting, specimen handling, and interpretation for each of these reasons.

We hope that the monograph fulfills a need for a practical guideline for intraoperative pathology consultation of the genitourinary specimens. We also hope it facilitates accurate diagnosis and effective communications with the clinical colleagues, who trust us with the task of guiding their surgical hands.

Houston, TX

Luan D. Truong
Steven S. Shen
Jae Y. Ro

Contents

Contributors

Ferran Algaba, M.D. Chief of Pathology Section, Fundació Puigvert, Associated Professor of Pathology, Morphological Department, Universitat Autónoma de Barcelona, Barcelona, Spain

Richard A. Goldfarb, M.D., F.A.C.S. Clinical Professor, Departments of Urology, Baylor College of Medicine, Houston, TX, USA; and The Methodist Hospital, Houston, TX, USA; and Weill Medical College of Cornell University, New York, NY, USA

Seth P. Lerner, M.D. Professor of Urology, Beth and Dave Swalm Chair in Urologic Oncology, Scott Department of Urology, Baylor College of Medicine, Houston, TX, USA

Jae Y. Ro, M.D., Ph.D. Professor, Departments of Pathology, The Methodist Hospital, Houston, TX, USA; and Weill Medical College of Cornell University, New York, NY, USA Adjunct Professor of Pathology, The University of Texas, MD Anderson Cancer Center, Houston, TX, USA

Steven S. Shen, M.D., Ph.D. Associate Professor, Departments of Pathology, The Methodist Hospital, Houston, TX, USA; and Weill Medical College of Cornell University, New York, NY, USA

Luan D. Truong, M.D. Professor, Departments of Pathology, The Methodist Hospital Houston, TX, USA; and Weill Medical College of Cornell University, New York, NY, USA; Adjunct Professor of Pathology and Medicine, Baylor College of Medicine, Houston, TX, USA

Chapter 1
Kidney

Luan D. Truong, Jae Y. Ro, Ri chard A.Go ldfarb,
andS teven S. Shen

REASONS FOR INTRAOPERATIVE PATHOLOGY CONSULTATION

Intraoperative pathology consultation (IPC) for kidney lesions is relatively infrequent.[1] However, it has a definite role in the surgical management of these lesions.[2] Gross and frozen section (FS) consultations were requested in 10.8% and 12.2%, respectively, for 6,907 radical nephrectomy specimens; whereas the percentages were 11.2% and 53.8%, respectively, for 600 partial nephrectomy specimens.[2] The possible reasons for intraoperative pathology consultation are listed in Table 1.1. The indications for IPC are not well defined and probably reflect personal preference, institutional tradition, and the types of hospitals.[2]

GROSS CONSULTATION

Clinical Background

Request from the surgeon to confirm the presence of a renal tumor is the most frequent type of gross consultation.[2] Most renal tumors are clinically assumed to be renal cell carcinoma (RCC) and are treated by radical nephrectomy, a decision mainly derived from clinical and imaging findings rather than from a tissue diagnosis. Usually only gross consultation is requested to confirm the lesion in the radical nephrectomy specimen. FS diagnosis of the tumor is usually not needed since it does not alter the type of surgical treatment. Gross consultation is also often requested for a predominantly hilar tumor to see whether it is urothelial carcinoma, for which the surgical treatment is different from RCC (*see also* Urothelial Carcinoma below).

1

L.D. Truong et al., *Frozen Section Library: Genitourinary Tract,*
Frozen Section Library 2, DOI 10.1007/978-1-4419-0691-5_1,
© Springer Science + Business Media, LLC 2009

TABLE 1.1 Reasons for intraoperative consultation for 325 consecutive renal specimens (materials from the Methodist Hospital and VA Medical Center, Houston, Texas).

Gross consultation	62%
Gross identification of renal or pelvic mass in the nephrectomy specimens	62%
Frozen section consultation	38%
Definitive diagnosis for a renal mass	5%
Diagnosis of a solid renal mass in unusual clinical or radiological settings	7%
Clinically suspected urothelial carcinoma and ureteral surgical margin	3%
Diagnosis of a cystic renal mass	5%
Surgical margin and diagnosis for tumors removed by partial nephrectomy	8%
Diagnosis of multiple renal masses	2%
Diagnosis of extrarenal masses or enlarged lymph nodes during nephrectomy	5%
Check for glomeruli in medical renal biopsies	1%
Status of kidneys donated for transplantation	3%

Specimen Handling

The submitted specimen is usually radical nephrectomy specimen. This specimen usually includes kidney, perirenal adipose tissue, Gerota fascia, renal pelvis, and a portion of ureter of variable length. Adrenal gland may or may not be included. We recommend the following way to handle a radical nephrectomy specimen. The intact specimen should be initially inspected for the blood vessels (usually marked with a tie or a metal clip by surgeons in the operating room) at the renal sinus for possible tumor thrombus, followed by identification of an usually short segment of ureter included in the specimen, which should be probed up to the pyelocalyceal system. The specimen is then bivalved through the renal pelvis guided by the ureteral probe for an accurate exposing of the renal sinus with the pyelocalyceal system, the renal parenchyma and the cut surface of the tumor. For an eccentric lesion, the original cut may not suffice, but additional cuts parallel to the original or perpendicular to the original sections should provide gross details. Peeling off the perinephric fat or bivalving the kidney from the perinephric side should be avoided since the relationship of the tumor and adjacent structures and perirenal fat invasion by the tumor may be distorted and cannot be accurately evaluated.

Interpretation

The above approach often clearly reveals the renal lesion with its cut surface as well as its relationship to the adjacent renal parenchyma, renal pelvis, renal sinus, and perirenal soft tissue. As a general rule, the location of the tumor, its gross appearance, and its tinctorial characteristics can often suggest the histological type, even without FS (Table 1.2). The epicenter of the tumor is particularly helpful for the differential diagnoses of tumors that involve predominantly the renal medulla/renal pyelocalyceal area. Tumors in this area raise the question of collecting duct carcinoma and high-grade urothelial carcinoma involving the renal medullary parenchyma. Not uncommonly, large tumors in this area may extend into the soft tissue in the renal sinus, and may involve the renal hilar vessels. The relationship of the tumor to the pyelocalyceal wall should be noted. Low-grade urothelial carcinomas typically appear as shaggy thickening of pelvic wall with protrusion of the tumor into the pelvic lumen (Fig. 1.1).

Gross observation to evaluate all the surgical margins (soft tissue, vascular, and ureteral) for tumor involvement should be done first. Submission of tissue for FS evaluation for these margins will vary depending on the opinion of the surgeon or the pathologist. It is usually not requested since involvement of these margins is very rare and in such case, the margin involvement is usually obvious intraoperatively as well as grossly.

If RCC is confirmed microscopically, additional surgery is usually not performed. However, if urothelial carcinoma is diagnosed, resection of the rest of the ureter with a cuff of bladder wall (nephrourerectomy) will be performed, and the surgeon may request FS for the distal surgical margin of this specimen (*see below*).

FROZEN SECTION TO ESTABLISH A DEFINITIVE DIAGNOSIS OF A RENAL MASS

Clinical Background

Most large and centrally located solid renal tumors are assumed to be RCC and are treated by radical nephrectomy, usually followed by a gross consultation.[3] FS is, however, sometimes requested for the following reasons: (1) To confirm the surgeon's clinical impression and provide the surgeon with additional information about the nature of the tumor for an informative discussion with the patient's family immediately after surgery; (2) To facilitate the decision on nodal dissection.

TABLE 1.2 Differential diagnosis of histological types of renal cell carcinoma.

	Gross features	Frozen section features
Clear cell	Well circumscribed with pseudocapsule; protruding from the renal cortex; variegated cut surface (solid, cystic, myxoid, hemorrhagic); bright yellow areas corresponding to the clear tumor cells; white tan areas corresponding to granular tumor cells	Cells with clear cytoplasm, low nuclear grade, well-defined cell membrane, forming sheets, nests, tubules, acini, ill-defined papillary fronds, and cysts containing red blood cells or eosinophilic fluid, separated by thin-walled blood vessels. Sometimes admixed with cells with granular eosinophilic cytoplasm and higher nuclear grade
Papillary	Well circumscribed with a fibrous capsule; usually confined to the kidney parenchyma; more often multifocal than other types; variegated cut surface, yellow (due to abundant macrophages within tumor), gray-tan, brown; often cystic/hemorrhagic	*Type 1*: Papillary and tubular structures lined by cells with rather scant, partially clear or granular cytoplasm, and low-grade nuclei; macrophages often within the papillary cores *Type 2*: Predominantly papillary structures lined by cells with more abundant eosinophilic cytoplasm, and higher nuclear grade, large nucleoli, without abundant macrophages in the papillary cores
Chromophobe	Well circumscribed; solid homogeneous tan to brown cut surface; focal hemorrhage or necrosis, or central scar in few cases	Three cell types: cells with abundant finely reticulated cytoplasm; cells with less abundant granular eosinophilic cytoplasm, with or without perinuclear halo; all with well-defined cell membrane; often low nuclear grade, irregular nuclear contour, and binucleation; forming solid or trabecular growth separated by thick-walled blood vessels (vs thin-walled blood vessels in clear cell RCC)

Collecting duct	Small tumor usually at medulla; larger tumor at any location; usually large tumor, gray white firm cut surface; indistinct border, often widespread invasion (adrenal gland, perirenal fat, renal sinus, renal pelvis)	Cells with amphophilic cytoplasm, large highly atypical nuclei; prominent nucleoli; forming complex tubulopapillary structures, microcysts with intracystic papillation; constant desmoplastic stroma; extensive infiltration of renal parenchyma; sometimes cytoplasmic mucin; sometimes carcinoma in situ in collecting ducts
Sarcomatoid	Sarcomatoid changes reflect in focal firm, white tan areas, against the background of one of the four above RCC types. The whole tumor may appears that way in case the sarcomatoid component overgrows and obliterates the parental RCC	Spindle or rarely round cells, atypical nuclei; different patterns, e.g., fibrosarcomatous, malignant fibrous histiocytomatous, undifferentiated; rarely heterologous sarcomatous components; often associated with the parental RCC

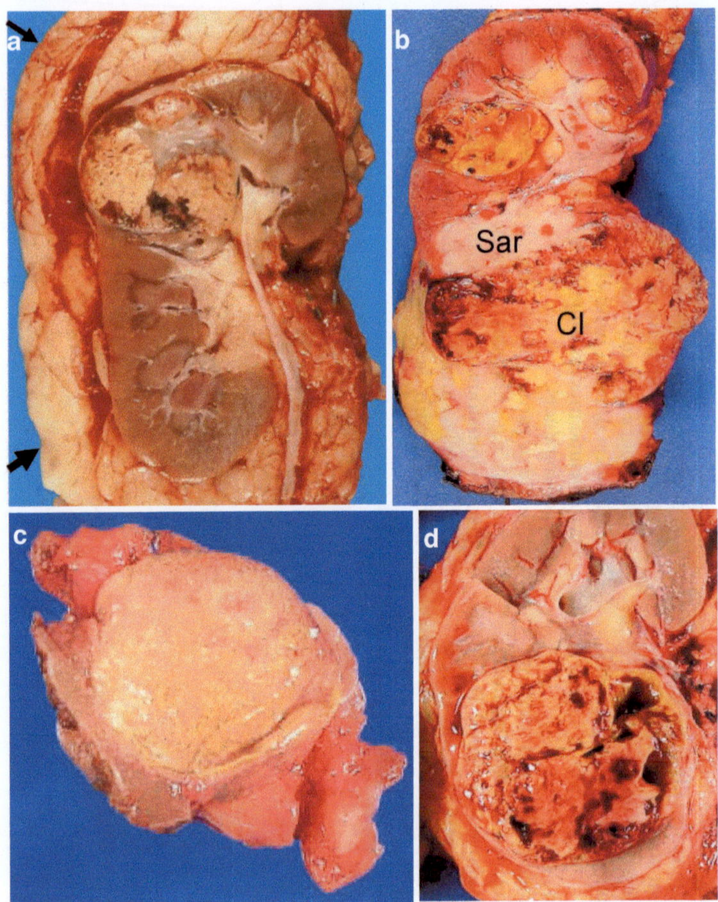

FIGURE 1.1 *Gross appearance of RCC.* (**a**) *Clear cell RCC.* Radical nephrectomy specimen bivalved to show ureter, pyelocalyceal system, renal sinus, kidney, tumor, perirenal adipose tissue, and fascia of Gerota (*arrows*); this fascia encases the specimen but is not grossly apparent due to its thinness. The tumor shows brightly yellow areas, with focal hemorrhagic, cystic, or myxoid changes. (**b**) *Sarcomatoid RCC* [white tan areas (Sar)] arising from a clear cell RCC (Cl). (**c**) *Papillary RCC, type 1* (partial nephrectomy): Circumscribed solid homogeneous tan cut surface. (**d**) *Papillary RCC, type 2:* Encapsulated tumor with yellowish solid areas and cystic changes.

Some features of the primary RCC (high stage, high nuclear grade, large size, a sarcomatoid component, and histological tumor necrosis) may indicate a higher chance of nodal metastasis.

FS may be requested in this context[4]; and (3) To establish a definite diagnosis for a solid renal mass with clinical or imaging features that are unusual for RCC. In the latter situation, lesions other than RCC are not infrequent and, in our experience, may include malakoplakia, xanthogranulomatous pyelonephritis (XGP), renal lymphoma, metastatic tumor, angiomyolipoma (AML), large renal medullary fibroma, leiomyoma, perirenal mesothelial cyst, subcapsular hematoma, adrenal cortical carcinoma extending to kidney, or mixed epithelial and stromal tumor of the kidney[3]; (4) To confirm the diagnosis of renal pelvic urothelial carcinoma, for which excision of the rest of the ureter is indicated (*see below*); (5) To establish a definitive diagnosis of a renal mass, which may dictate the choice among conservative treatment, partial nephrectomy, or radical nephrectomy[5]; and (6) To confirm the involvement of the surgical margins (which is exceptional).

Specimen Handling

The handling is similar to those submitted for gross consultation (*see above*). After the cut surface of the lesion is examined, areas of different gross appearance should be sampled for FS. Attention should be paid to avoid necrotic or hemorrhagic area when choosing tissue for FS.

Interpretation

Discussed below are selected differential diagnostic problems derived from our experience or literature.

The Diagnosis of RCC and Its Histological Subtypes

The 2004 WHO classification recognizes five major types of RCC: clear cell, papillary, chromophobe, collecting duct, and unclassified RCC. Sarcomatoid RCC is not considered a specific histological type and is regarded as a dedifferentiated element of one of these above types, since the sarcomatoid component can be seen in all the above recognizable histological types of RCC.[6] Each of these types of RCC has characteristic features that enable an accurate diagnosis by gross examination alone or combined with FS (Table 1.2 and Figs. 1.1–1.10). Since RCC displays a broad morphological spectrum and there are unclassified RCCs as well as hybrid tumors (two or more recognizable cell types), its histological classification on FS diagnosis may not be possible in some cases. Deferment on histological typing in these cases is appropriate and does not impact patient care. Histological typing of RCC is usually not a

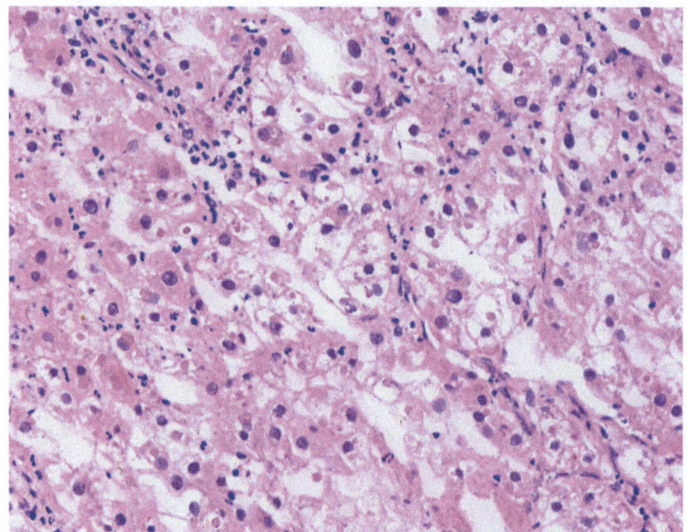

FIGURE 1.2 *Clear cell RCC, high nuclear grade*. Typical tumor cells with abundant granular, clear, or mixed cytoplasm, and large nuclei. Stromal vascularity may not be obvious.

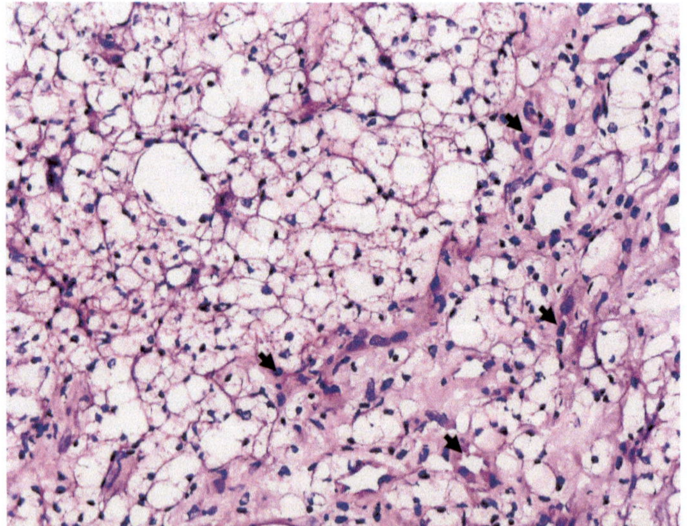

FIGURE 1.3 *Clear cell RCC, low nuclear grade*. Tumor cells with small hyperchromatic nuclei, abundant clear cytoplasm, and well-defined cell border. Prominent stromal vascularity (*arrows*) is characteristic.

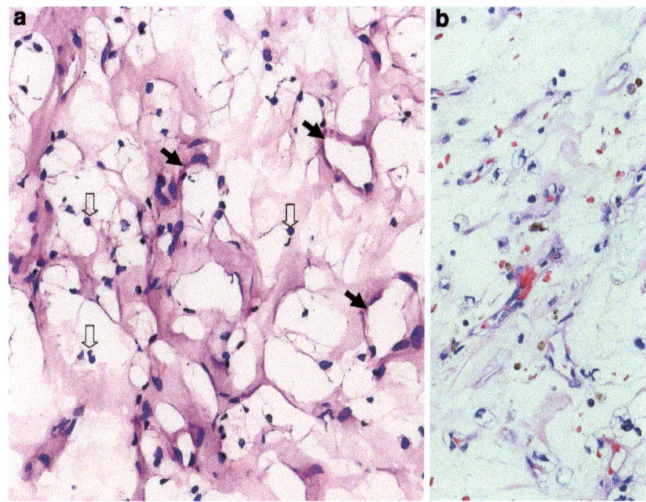

FIGURE 1.4 *Clear cell RCC, low grade.* (**a**) The tumor may be composed mostly of areas with abundant thin-walled blood vessels with prominent endothelial cells (*solid arrows*). Isolated tumor cells may be present (*open arrows*) but are not obvious in FS. This type of stroma strongly suggests the diagnosis of clear cell RCC. (**b**) The corresponding permanent section shows isolated tumor cells with clear cytoplasm.

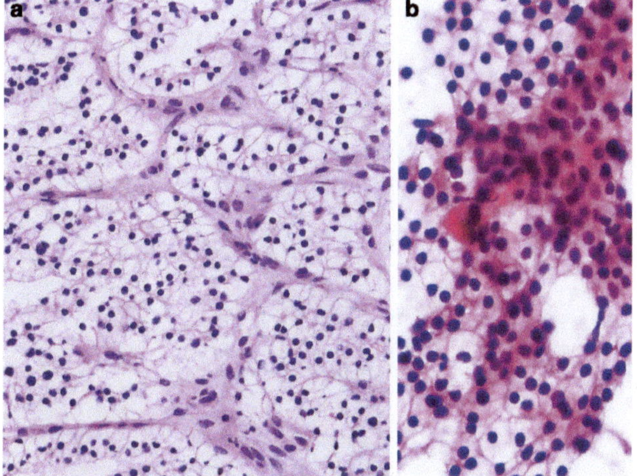

FIGURE 1.5 *Clear cell RCC, low grade.* FS (**a**) and touch prep (**b**). Fixation in formalin, rather than alcohol, and longer staining with hematoxylin enhance the cell membrane and the clear appearance of the cytoplasm.

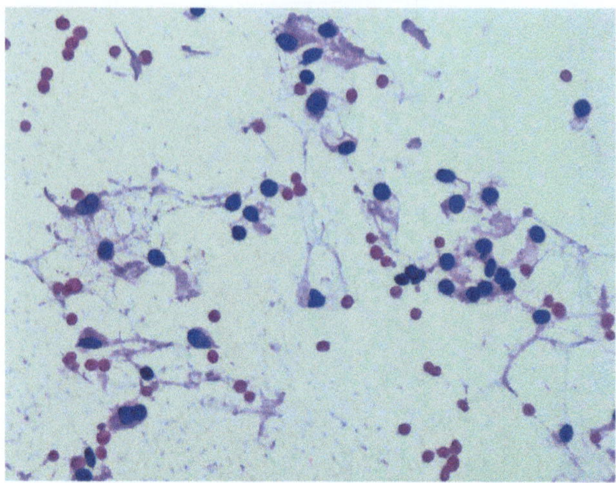

FIGURE 1.6 *Clear cell RCC, low grade.* In touch prep, the tumor cells may appear as bare hyperchromatic nuclei with artifactual loss of the clear cytoplasm. This artifact, which is quite frequent for the cystic variant, is characteristic for low-grade clear cell RCC and should suggest the diagnosis.

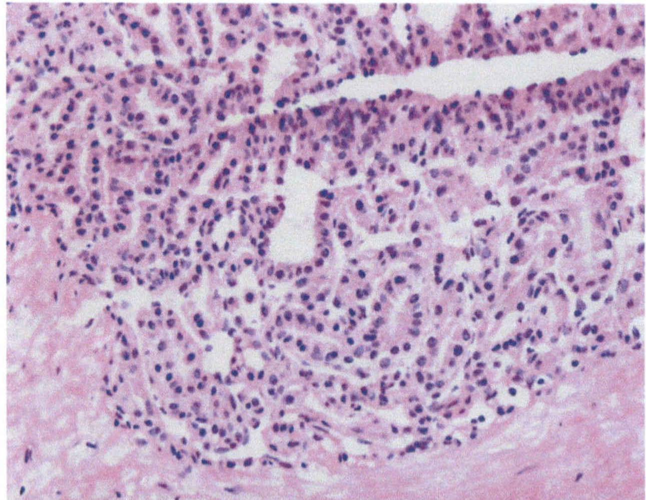

FIGURE 1.7 *Papillary RCC, type 1.* The tumor is encapsulated. In spite of the name, it can be composed mostly of tubules, as seen here. The tumor cells typically display low nuclear atypia, and scant cytoplasm.

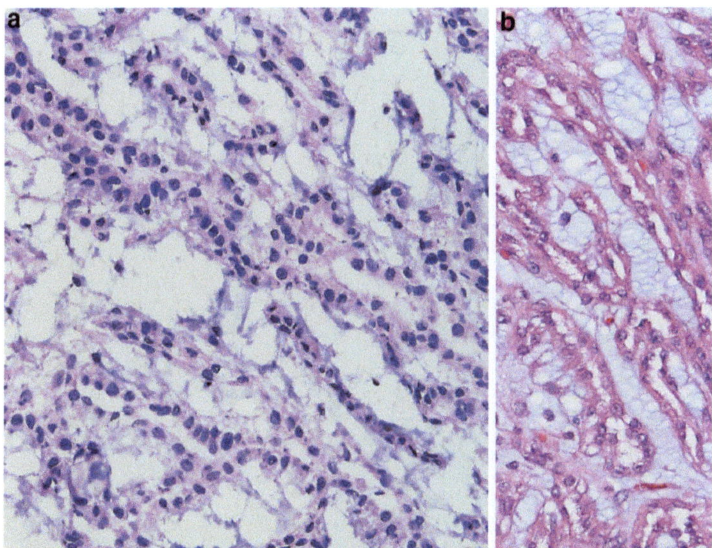

FIGURE 1.8 *Mucinous spindle and tubular cell carcinoma.* (**a**) The tumor cells display low nuclear grade and scant cytoplasm forming tubules, which can simulate papillary RCC, type 1. The stromal mucin is characteristic, but as shown here, may be inconspicuous in FS. (**b**) The corresponding permanent section displays typical features including abundant stromal mucin.

determinant for intraoperative treatment and RCC typing is usually not requested by the surgeon. Nevertheless, one should be familiar with the gross and FS spectrum of various RCC histological types to facilitate their identification and rule out potential mimickers.

The features of RCC histological types in FS reflect their morphological spectrum in permanent sections (Table 1.2 and Figs. 1.1–1.10). FS may create artifacts, leading to diagnostic dilemma. Touch preparation often provides excellent cytological features of tumor cells, complementary to FS (Figs. 1.1–1.10).

Differential Diagnoses of Clear Cell RCC, XGP, and Malakoplakia

Although these entities may show subtle imaging or gross differences among them (Table 1.3 and Figs. 1.11 and 1.15), a definitive diagnosis usually requires FS. An FS diagnosis depends on recognizing the cell type characteristic for each entity.[7,8] The clear cells in solid areas

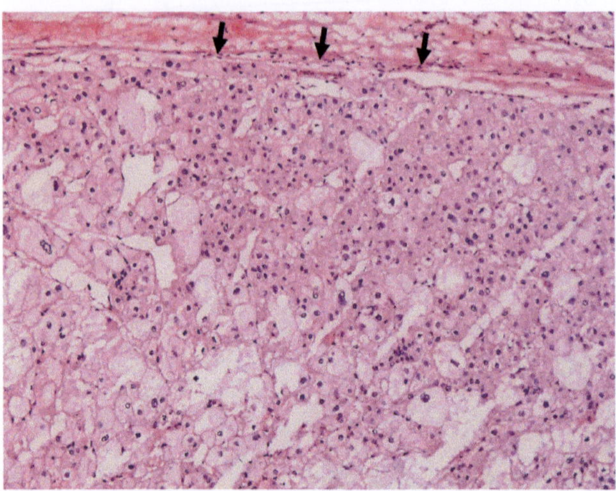

FIGURE 1.9 *Chromophobe RCC*. This field shows all three different cell types (reticular, eosinophilc with perinuclear halo, and eosinophilic without perinuclear halo; *see also* Fig. 1.10) described in chromophobe RCC, but one type may dominate in an individual tumor. Tumor encapsulation (*arrows*) and well-defined cell membrane are characteristic.

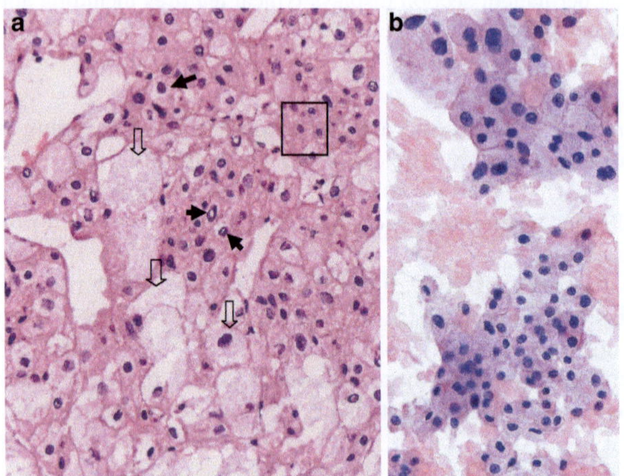

FIGURE 1.10 *Chromophobe RCC*. (**a**) Characteristic features: Three cell types [reticular with abundant cytoplasm (*open arrows*), eosinophilic with perinuclear halo (*solid arrows*), or without perinuclear halo (*square*)], well-defined cell membrane, and irregular nuclear contour. (**b**) Several of these features are seen in touch prep.

TABLE 1.3 Clear cell renal cell carcinoma (*RCC*) vs xanthogranulomatous pyelonephritis (*XGP*) vs renal malakoplakia.

	Gross	Microscopic
RCC	Well circumscribed, yellow cut surface with focal hemorrhagic, necrotic or myxomatous degeneration; +/− perirenal extension; renal parenchyma and pyelocalyceal system usually normal	Clear or clear/granular cells in sheets, with little or no intervening fibrosis or chronic inflammation. Solid, alveolar, cystic, pseudopapillary growth patterns; prominent anastomosing complex vascular stroma
XGP	Rarely circumscribed, often diffuse and poorly demarcated; yellow and white variegated cut surface with often fibroinflammatory changes; constant extension to perirenal or peripelvic soft tissue; renal parenchyma usually atrophic; frequent distortion of the pyelocalyceal system	Sheets of "xanthoma" cells with fine vacuolated cytoplasm admixed with fibrosis, chronic, and acute inflammation
Malakoplakia	Similar to XGP	Sheets of von Hanssemann cells with diagnostic Michaelis-Guttmann bodies; with or without admixed fibrosis and chronic and/or acute inflammation

of RCC usually appear intact with preserved cell membrane and characteristic clear or clear/granular cytoplasm separated by a rich vascular network recognizable in FS (Figs. 1.2–1.6). Difficulty may be encountered when the delicate cytoplasm of the tumor cells disintegrates and results in bare nuclei (Figs. 1. 4 and 1.6); this is especially true for low-grade tumor cells from cystic areas. Alternatively, during FS, the "clear" cytoplasm of tumor cells may display a faint eosinophilia. Fixing the frozen tissue sections in formalin for 1 min and routine staining but with longer staining with hematoxylin (2 min) can better delineate the cell membrane and accentuate the clear cytoplasm (Fig. 1.5).[9] The features of clear cells can be also well recognized in touch preparation (Figs. 1.5 and 1.6).

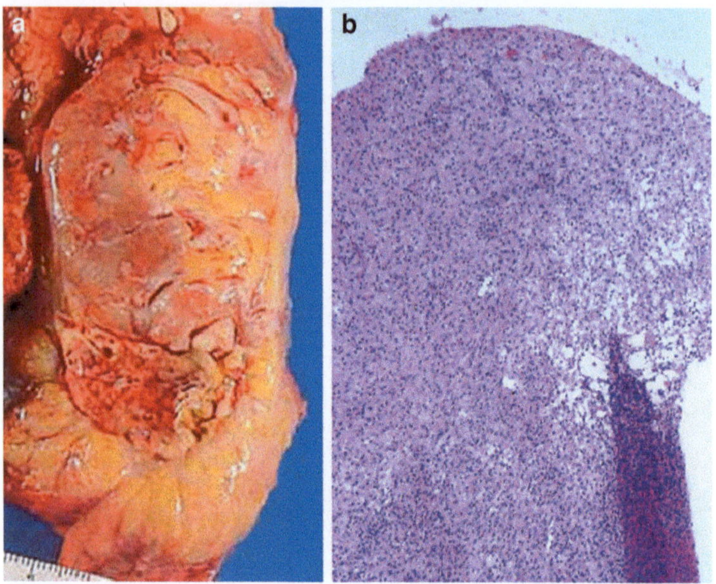

FIGURE 1.11 *Xanthogranulomatous Pyelonephritis*. (**a**) Brightly yellowish partially cystic mass, with perinephric involvement, closely simulating a clear cell RCC. (**b**) Cellular mass lesion with a clear cell area in the right.

The xanthomatous cells of XGP, instead of having a clear cytoplasm, typically display abundant and *finely vacuolated cytoplasm*, which can be recognized in FS. They are often associated with other inflammatory cells (Figs. 1.12 and 1.13). Spindle cells, potentially simulating spindle cell tumors, may be a major component in organized XGP. Residual macrophages admixed with inflammatory cells should raise this possibility (Fig. 1.14). Small clusters of xanthoma cells are frequent in papillary RCC and should not cause diagnostic problem; however, a rare case of papillary RCC may have confluent, grossly visible sheets of xanthoma cells, which can be misleading on FS.[10] In such a situation, careful evaluation of the FS for an epithelial component is necessary.

The von Hanssemann histiocytes typical for malakoplakia may closely simulate RCC cells, especially the granular cells; however, many of these cells contain the pathognomonic Michaelis-Guttmann bodies. In a few cases of malakoplakia personally encountered, the Michaelis-Guttmann bodies, for unknown reason, are deeply basophilic in FS and much easier to recognize in this context than in permanent sections (Figs. 1.15 and 1.16).

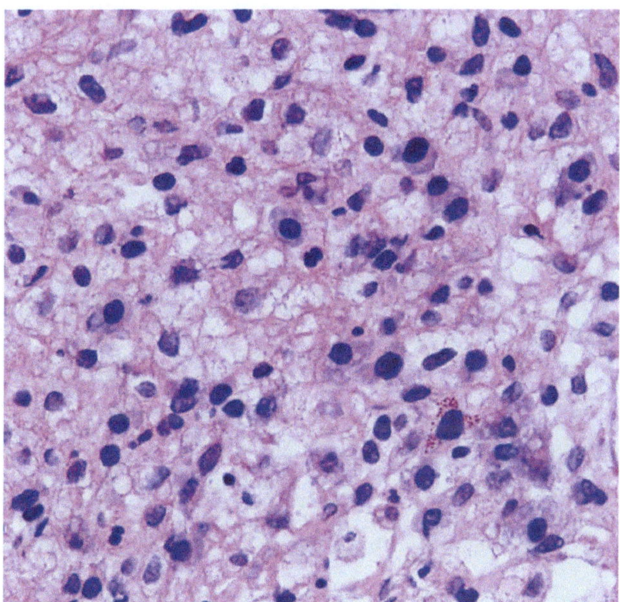

FIGURE 1.12 *Xanthogranulomatous Pyelonephritis*. Xanthoma cells with clear/vacuolated/granular cytoplasm, simulating RCC clear cells. Stromal vascularity, typical for clear cell RCC, is not present. This is a diagnostic clue.

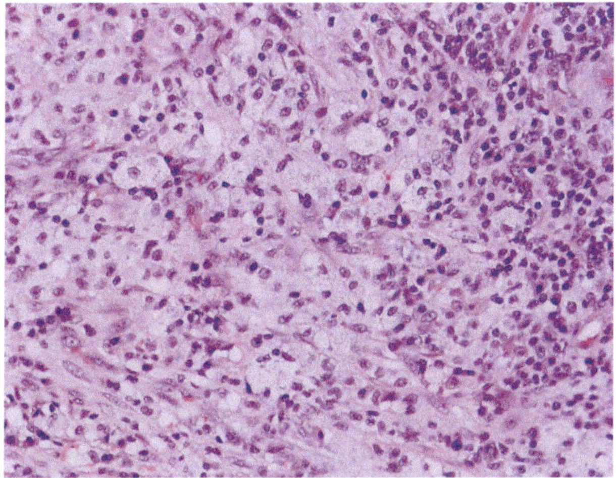

FIGURE 1.13 *Xanthogranulomatous pyelonephritis*. Aggregated xanthoma cells, simulating RCC clear cells. These cells are admixed with inflammatory cells, a diagnostic clue.

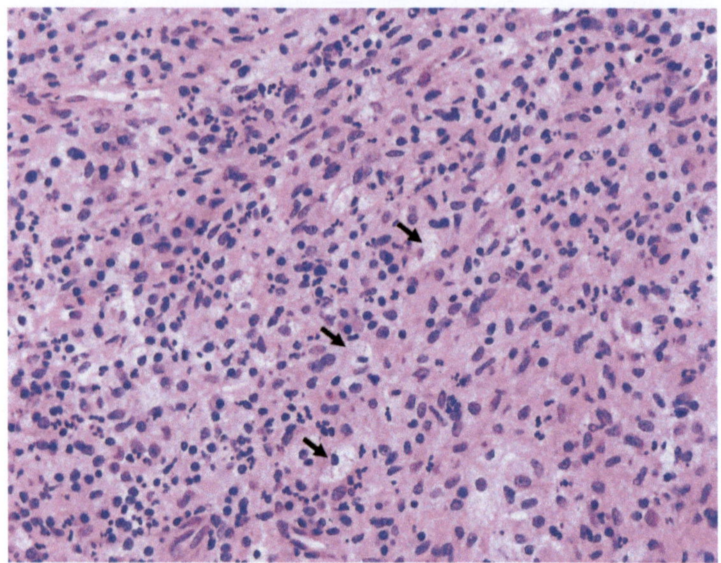

FIGURE 1.14 *Xanthogranulomatous pyelonephritis*. A focal hypercellular area with spindle cells, potentially simulating spindle cell tumors, including sarcomatoid RCC. Residual macrophages (*arrows*) and admixed inflammation should raise the possibility of inflammatory lesions including organized XGP.

Oncocytoma and Chromophobe RCC

These two tumors need to be separated since oncocytoma is benign whereas chromophobe RCC is a carcinoma that is often low grade but may behave aggressively.[11-13] Intraoperative recognition of these tumors is irrelevant in case of total nephrectomy, but may be important in a partial nephrectomy specimen where the margin is critical for a chromophobe carcinoma. FS is needed since their gross appearance can be very similar (Fig. 1.17). Features that help separate them are listed in Table 1.4. Two histological subtypes of chromophobe RCC are recognized, that is typical and eosinophilic.[13] Typical chromophobe RCC can often be separated from oncocytoma by the features listed in Table 1.4 and illustrated in Figs. 1.17–1.20. During FS, the perinuclear halo and/or the well-defined cell membrane typical for chromophobe RCC may not be obvious in tissue sections, especially in suboptimal preparation. However, these features may be better appreciated in touch preparations (Fig. 1.10). The characteristic growth pattern of chromophobe RCC, that is closely packed broad sheets of

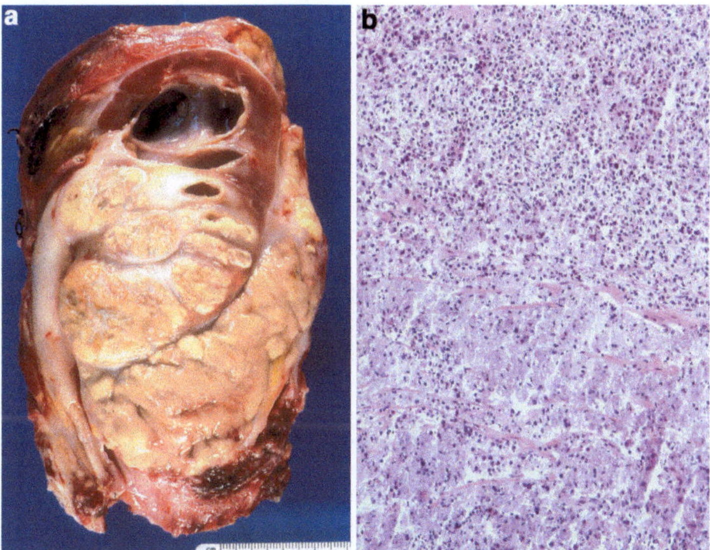

FIGURE 1.15 *Malakoplakia*. (**a**) Renal mass with multinodular brightly yellow cut surface and perinephric extension, simulating clear cell RCC. (**b**) At low magnification, the mass is composed of aggregated cells with variable but often abundant eosinophilic cytoplasm (von Hanssemann cells). Inflammatory cells are not obvious in this case, but can be pronounced in malakoplakia. Prominent stromal vascularity, typical for RCC, is not seen.

tumor cells and abundant cytoplasm, remains helpful since it is maintained in FS and is not seen in oncocytoma (Fig. 1.8). Many of the features that are characteristic for typical chromophobe RCC and help separate it from oncocytoma are not obvious in the eosinophilic variant of chromophobe RCC. Differentiation of this variant from oncocytoma remains problematic, even in permanent sections.[13] The diagnosis of oncocytic renal neoplasm with deferment to permanent sections is appropriate in this situation.

Angiomyolipoma

The utility of FS in the surgical management of angiomyolipoma (AML) is well documented.[14] Accurate FS diagnosis of AML is important since it is rather frequent and can attain large size, but is almost uniformly benign and is being increasingly considered as a good candidate for partial nephrectomy.[15] Indeed, the frequency of benign renal tumors in partial nephrectomy specimens (up to 34%) is higher than that in total nephrectomy specimens (about 10%),[16] and this increase is chiefly due to AML and oncocytoma. In the context

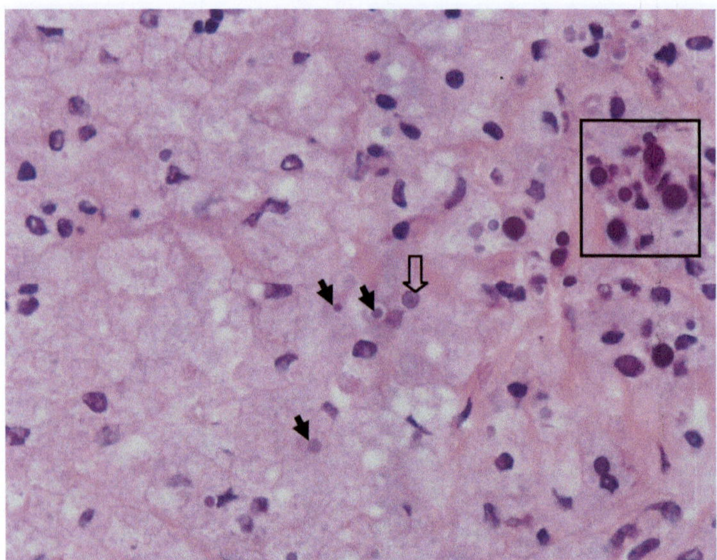

FIGURE 1.16 *Malakoplakia*. Different forms of the diagnostic Michaelis-Guttmann bodies, including basophilic bodies without internal structure (*solid arrows*), with lamellar appearance (*open arrows*) or with calcification (*square*). These bodies are more apparent in FS than in permanent sections, probably due to their more basophilia in the FS.

of laparoscopic partial nephrectomy specimen, if tumor tissue is identified at the surgical margin and if it is malignant, immediate total nephrectomy is usually considered; however, this procedure may not be indicated if the tumor is benign, as in AML.[17,18]

Since AML is composed of adipose tissue, smooth muscle, and blood vessels in various proportions, it has been confused with many other renal tumors during FS.[3,17,18] Imaging study can accurately identify AML if it is composed mostly of adipose tissue, but remains problematic if the other components predominate.[19] *In our experience, touch preparation of AML may not facilitate the diagnosis and may even be misleading since the tumor cell clusters closely simulate those of RCC.* Note that the three components of AML in tissue sections remain essential for diagnosis (Fig. 1.21). The adipose tissue component may display severe frozen artifacts and appear as variably sized and ragged clear spaces interspersed between spindled cells and vessels (Figs. 1.21–1.23). This artifact, however, has a diagnostic value since, in our experience, it is regularly seen and should raise the possibility of AML. One important

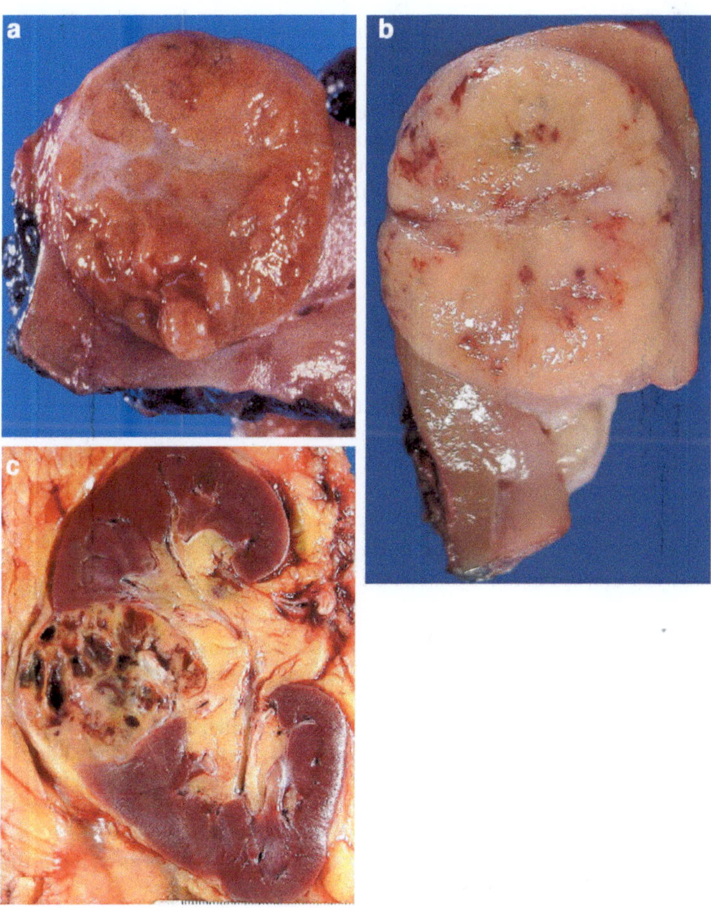

FIGURE 1.17 (**a**) *Oncocytoma*: Encapsulated mass, with a mahogany brown cut surface and a central scar, without necrotic/cystic changes. (**b**) *Chromophobe RCC*: Similar cut surface as oncocytoma, but more tan with a few areas of hemorrhage. (**c**) *Chromophobe RCC:* This tumor has more cystic/hemorrhagic changes. These changes are often not seen in oncocytoma.

clue for a correct diagnosis is abnormal thickened blood vessels with radial array of spindled cells around them (Figs. 1.21–1.23). This feature, characteristic for AML, is not seen in other renal tumors and can be readily appreciated in FS.[19]

AML may be composed predominantly of smooth muscle and vascular components, with significant nuclear atypia as noted in about 8% of AML or in the recently described epithelioid AML[19].

TABLE 1.4 Oncocytoma vs chromophobe renal cell carcinoma (*RCC*).

	Gross	Microscopic
Oncocytoma	Circumscribed, mahogany cut surface, +/− central scar, extrarenal extension rare, possible small hemorrhage, no obvious necrosis	Acini, tubules, small cysts, islands of tumor cells separated by edematous poorly cellular stroma, uniformly eosinophilic cytoplasm, uniform round nuclei, *cell membrane not well defined*, isolated highly atypical cells (5% of cases)
Chromophobe RCC, typical type	As above, but hemorrhage or necrosis possible	Predominantly sheets of tumor cells separated by scant vascularized stroma, abundant reticulated or eosinophilic cytoplasm with *perinuclear halo, well-defined cell membrane*, irregular nuclear contour, occasional binucleation
Chromophobe RCC, eosinophilic type	As the typical variant	Tubules or trabeculae separated by scant vascularized stroma; smaller cells with eosinophilic cytoplasm; cell membrane less well defined and perinuclear halo not as obvious as those of the classic type

This variant of AML can be confused with other renal tumors such as *high-grade RCC, sarcomatoid RCC, dedifferentiated retroperitoneal liposarcoma, primary renal sarcomas, inflammatory myofibroblastic tumor* (*inflammatory pseudotumor*), or *large cell lymphoma*. A correct FS diagnosis should be achieved by always considering AML in the differential diagnoses of an unusual renal tumor and by recognizing the characteristic perivascular cell array mentioned above (Fig. 1.23). In contrast, sarcomatoid RCC is frequently associated with areas typical for other histological types of RCC recognized by gross or FS.[20] True renal sarcoma is very rare and practically is not a consideration. Other spindle cell tumors such as *leiomyoma, inflammatory myofibroblastic tumor,*

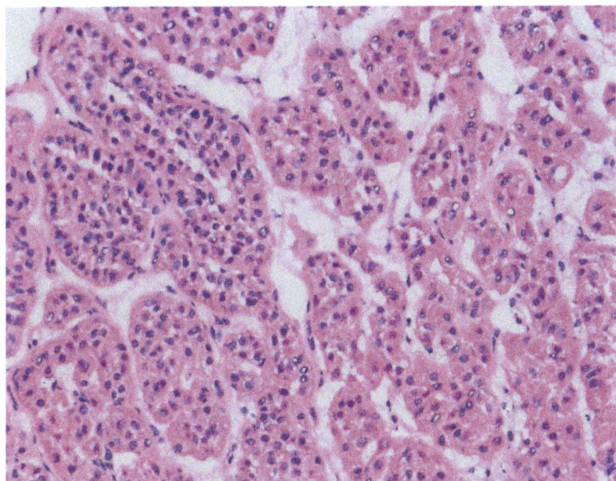

FIGURE 1.18 *Oncocytoma.* Tumor cells with abundant eosinophilic cytoplasm, round nuclei, inconspicuous cell membrane; forming islands, or trabeculae, separated by edematous paucicellular stroma. The tumor cells shown in the left side which have less cytoplasm ("oncoblasts") are characteristic for oncocytoma and may serve as a diagnostic clue.

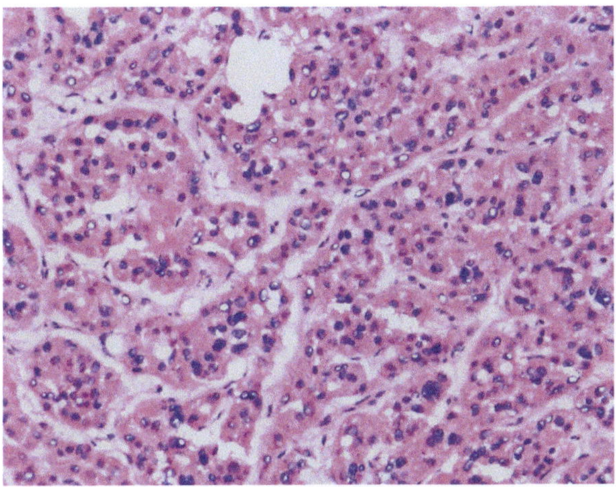

FIGURE 1.19 *Oncocytoma with cytological atypia.* An area with markedly atypical tumor cell nuclei, against a background of otherwise typical oncocytoma elsewhere. These focal changes are infrequent (about 5% of oncocytoma), but they are characteristic for oncocytoma and may even serve as a diagnostic clue. Oncocytoma with these changes remains benign.

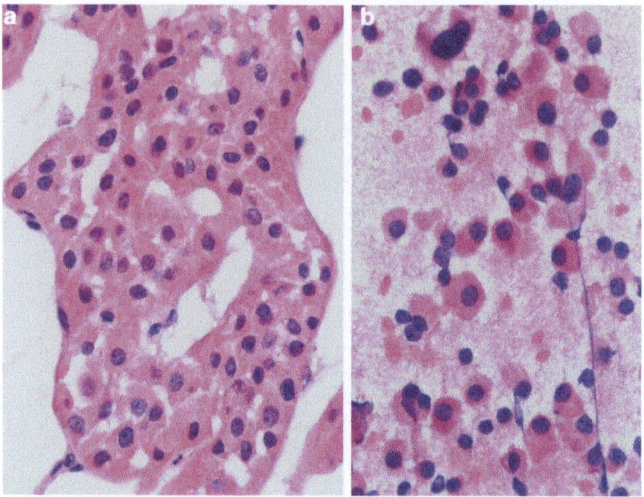

FIGURE 1.20 *Oncocytoma*. (**a**) Tumor cells with abundant eosinophilic cytoplasm, round nuclei, and inconspicuous cell membrane. (**b**) These cytological features are obvious in touch prep. Poor cohesiveness of tumor cells is also characteristic.

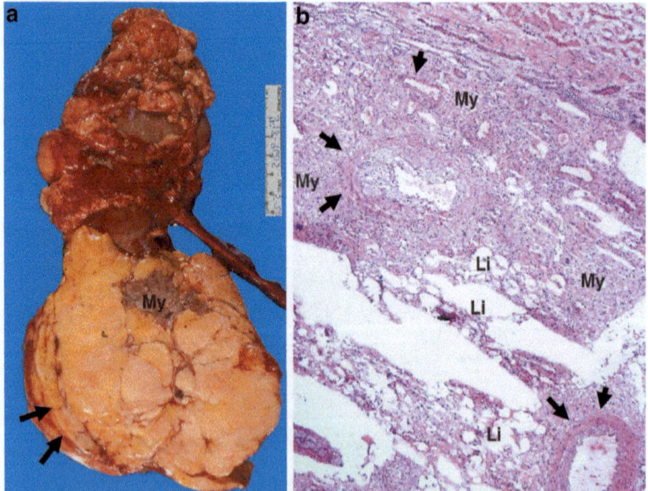

FIGURE 1.21 *Angiomyolipoma*. (**a**) A voluminous tumor with a predominantly extrarenal component, composed mostly of what appears as adipose tissue, with a small brownish area of myoid (*My*) component.

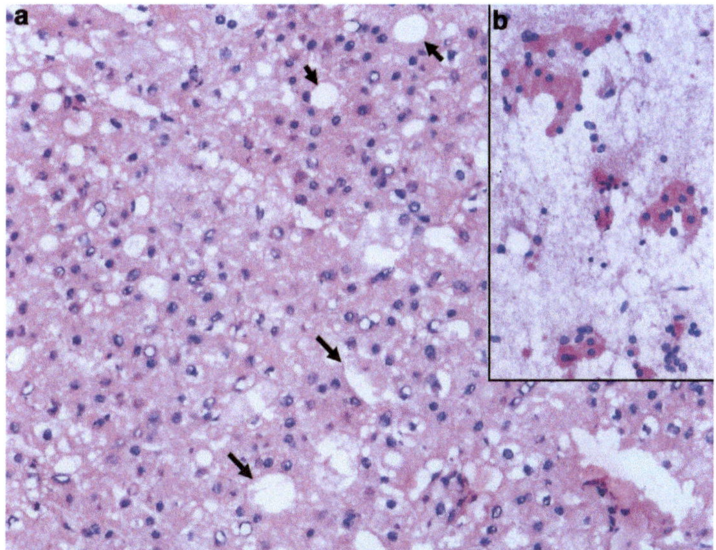

FIGURE 1.22 *Angiomyolipoma.* (**a**) The tumor may be composed almost entirely of the myoid component characterized by cells with abundant clear/vacuolated/granular cytoplasm, simulating RCC. The vascular component characteristic for angiomyolipoma may be inconspicuous in this variant of angiomyolipoma. A diagnostic clue includes clear spaces (*arrows*), which may appear as artifact, but indeed represent lipocytes. This should prompt angiomyolipoma as a diagnostic possibility and further FS sampling for other diagnostic features. (**b**) Touch prep is perhaps misleading since the myoid cells closely simulate cells from other renal cell tumor types.

and *solitary fibrous tumor* are both exceptional and their spindle cell component displays little or no atypia. *Mesoblastic nephroma* or *metanephric stromal tumor* features prominent spindled cells, but these cells are clearly benign and these two tumors are practically limited to the first few years of life.[21]

FIGURE 1.21 (continued) The tumor still respects the boundary of the Gerota's fascia (*arrows*), allowing excision of the tumor along the plane of this fascia, a feature not seen in retroperitoneal liposarcoma. (**b**) Three components may be seen: The myoid component (My) appearing as solid areas on lower magnification, the opened thick-walled blood vessels with apparent replacement of the adventitia by the myoid cells (*arrows*), and the lipomatous component which appears as artifactual clear spaces (*Li*). This artifact is, however, typical for angiomyolipoma and is a diagnostic clue. The presence of all three components is diagnostic for angiomyolipoma, but this may not be seen in every tumor.

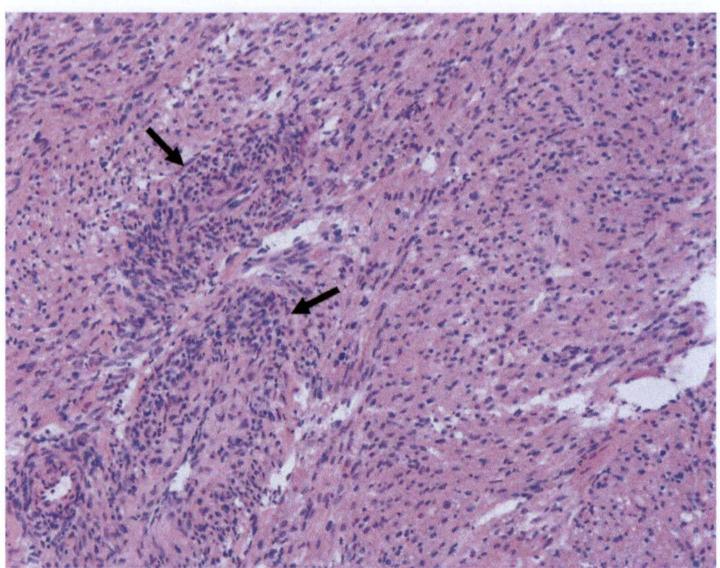

Figure 1.23 *Myoid-rich angiomyolipoma*: This tumor is composed almost entirely of ovoid or spindle cells, simulating other renal spindle cell tumors. However, the presence of large thick-walled blood vessels without adventitia (*arrows*) is diagnostic for angiomyolipoma. A peculiar increase in medial cellularity is also noted.

AML composed predominantly of adipose tissue may be confused with well-differentiated retroperitoneal liposarcoma; this is especially true when AML attains large size and consists of a large extrarenal component (Fig. 1.21).[19] The surgeon tends to be aware of the possibility of AML since, even in the above context, AML tends to respect the boundary of Gerota fascia, allowing the surgeon to excise the tumor along the natural tissue plane delineated by this fascia. This is not the case for bulky retroperitoneal liposarcoma. A correct FS diagnosis is also aided by an awareness of this type of AML, the presence of a constant, albeit small, intrarenal component, and microscopic fields of vascular/smooth muscle even in areas which grossly look like adipose tissue (Fig. 1.24).

FS can reveal AML tissue in renal vein or in other organs such as spleen, para-aortic lymph nodes, or liver, but these are considered multifocal disease rather than metastasis.[19,22]

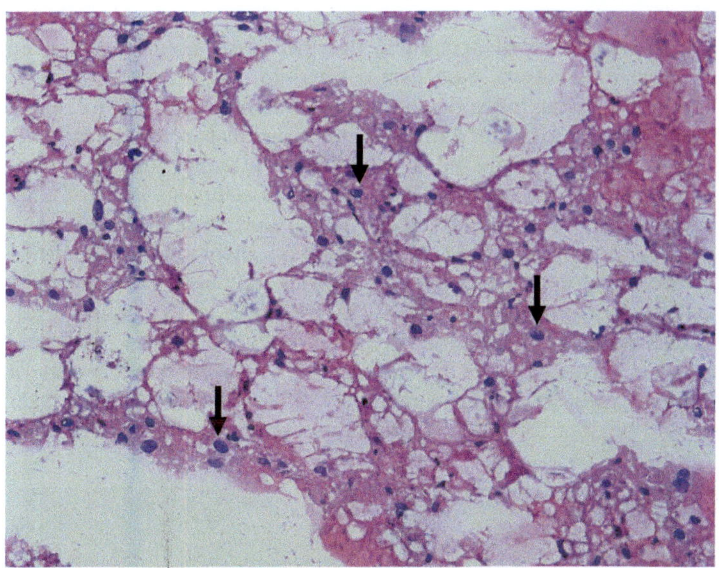

FIGURE 1.24 *Angiomyolipoma*: FS from a grossly "lipomatous" area shows numerous "artifactual" clear spaces, which in fact represent adipose tissue. In addition, few isolated myoid cells (*arrows*) are frequently seen in these areas and represent a diagnostic clue.

FROZEN SECTION FOR CLINICALLY SUSPECTED UROTHELIAL CARCINOMA AND URETER/BLADDER CUFF SURGICAL MARGIN

Clinical Background

If a preoperative diagnosis of renal pelvic urothelial carcinoma is made, the standard treatment is *nephroureterectomy*. This type of specimen may be submitted for confirmation of tumor grossly and FS of the distal surgical margin.

For a centrally located/hilar tumor in which urothelial carcinoma is clinically suspected but not preoperatively diagnosed, *nephrectomy* is usually performed and FS may be requested to confirm the diagnosis. This is important since the diagnosis of urothelial carcinoma mandates removal of the rest of the ureter together with a cuff of bladder wall to prevent tumor recurrence. FS evaluation of the distal surgical margin may also be requested since urothelial carcinoma is often multifocal and may involve this margin.

Specimen Handling

For the *nephrectomy* specimen, the specimen should be bivalved as described above. Successful bivalving of the nephrectomy specimen through the pyelocalyceal system is very helpful, since this often demonstrates in case of urothelial carcinoma that the tumor develops from the pyelocalyceal system, with or without invasion into the kidney (Fig. 1.25). FS diagnosis of urothelial carcinoma is also facilitated by noting that samples taken from the portion which invades kidney may not display typical features of urothelial carcinoma, but those from the pelvic portion of the same tumor often do.[23] (Figs. 1.25–1.28).

The *nephroureterectomy* specimen includes kidney, perirenal adipose tissue, Gerota fascia, the entire ureter, and a cuff of bladder wall. Bivalving the kidney and opening of the ureter should be done as for the nephrectomy specimen. FS to determine

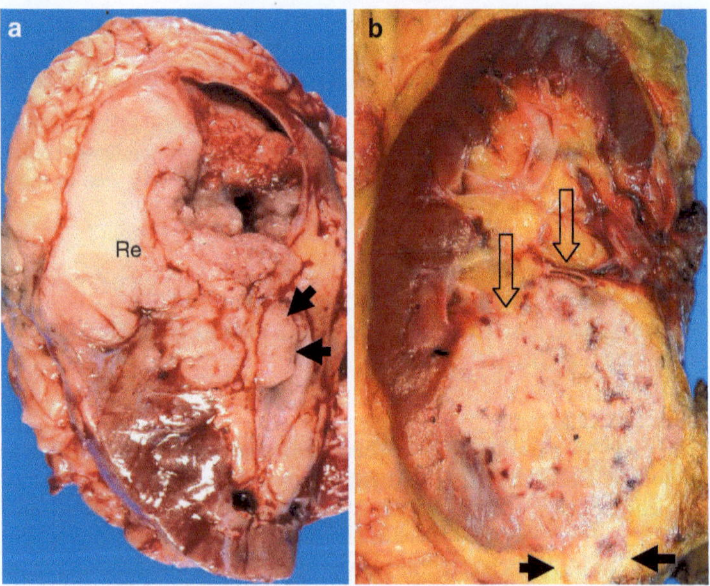

FIGURE 1.25 (a) *Urothelial carcinoma*: Bivalving the nephrectomy specimen through the pyelocalyceal system shows a tumor mass that involves the pelvic wall and pelvic lumen (*arrows*), together with a renal component (*Re*). The renal component may simulate other central/hilar renal tumors, but the pelvic component is characteristic for urothelial carcinoma and supports this diagnosis. (b) *Collecting duct RCC*: A large central/hilar mass with irregular border and multifocal involvement of both perirenal fat (*solid arrows*) and sinus fat (*open arrows*).

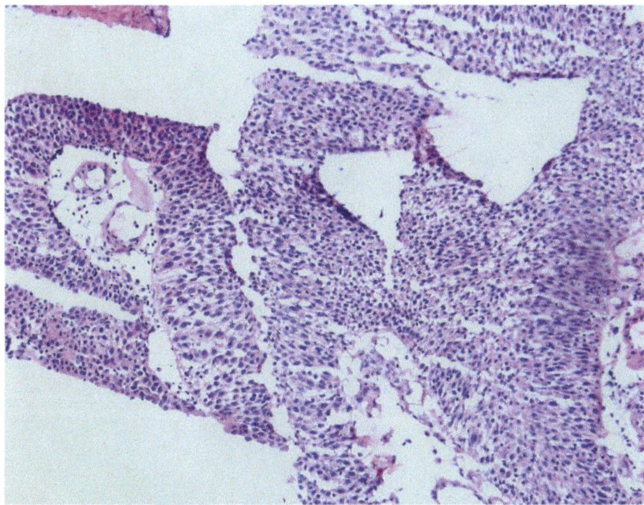

FIGURE 1.26 *Urothelial carcinoma*: Typical features, that is, multilayered atypical urothelial cells forming papillary structures, are seen in the tissue taken from the pelvic wall tumor in Fig. 1.25a.

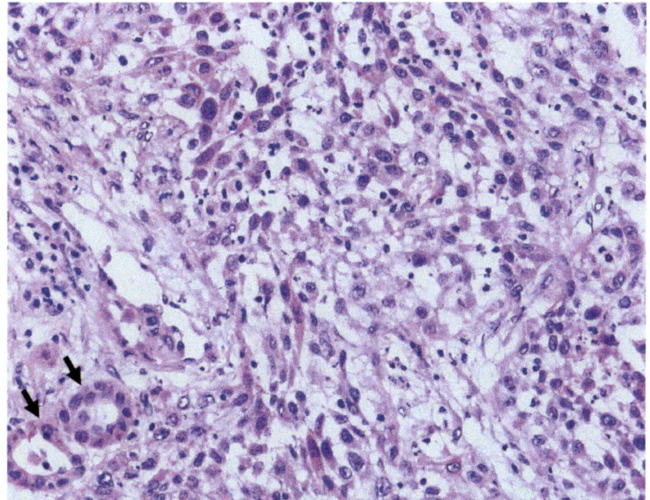

FIGURE 1.27 *Urothelial carcinoma*: Spindle and cuboidal cells not readily diagnostic for urothelial carcinoma in the tissue taken from the renal component of the tumor in Fig. 1.25a. Residual renal tubules are seen (*arrows*).

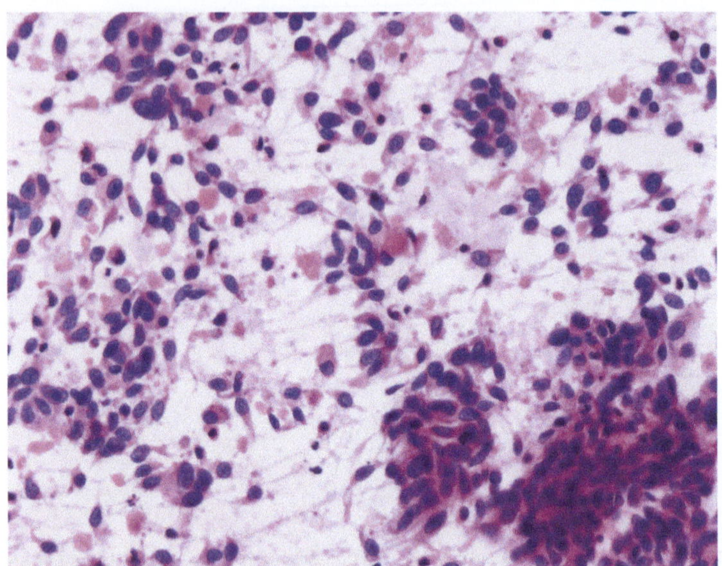

FIGURE 1.28 *Urothelial carcinoma*: In touch prep, the tumor cells typically display cuboidal or spindle shape cytoplasm with a "solid" eosinophilic appearance. They form papillary structures, small clusters, or isolated cells.

whether the distal surgical margin is involved by in situ or invasive urothelial neoplasm may be requested. The entire bladder cuff margin should be submitted. Whether tissue sampling should be circumferential (parallel to the surgical resection plan) or radial (perpendicular to the surgical resection plan) is probably optional, depending on the gross examination of the distal margin.

1.4.3. Interpretations

Urothelial carcinoma must be differentiated from other tumors, which may involve renal medulla predominantly or share some histological features with urothelial carcinoma. They include *collecting duct RCC*,[24,25] *primary renal pelvic adenocarcinoma*,[26] *metastatic adenocarcinoma*,[26] and *high-grade papillary RCC* (Table 1.5) This differential diagnosis can be problematic since urothelial carcinoma of renal pelvis is often of high grade (70%) and may display focal unusual growth patterns such as undifferentiated, micropapillary, spindle cell, clear cell, or gland-like formation (40%).[23]

Urothelial carcinoma may be confused with either papillary RCC or collecting duct RCC since papillary structures may predominate

Table 1.5 Differential diagnoses of renal pelvic urothelial carcinoma.

	Gross	Microscopic
Urothelial carcinoma	Tumor involvement of renal pelvic wall and lumen, +/– renal parenchymal extension, not encapsulated or circumscribed	Features of high- or low-grade urothelial carcinoma; squamous or glandular differentiation possible, but the urothelial carcinoma component always present. Features of urothelial carcinoma usually obvious in the pelvic component but less so in the renal invasive component; urothelial carcinoma in situ may be present
Collecting duct RCC	Tan white tumor mass predominantly in renal medulla, usually large tumor, gray white firm cut surface; indistinct border, often widespread invasion (adrenal gland, perirenal fat, renal sinus, renal pelvis)	Cells with amphophilic cytoplasm, large highly atypical nuclei; prominent nucleoli; forming complex tubulopapillary structures, microcysts with intracystic papillation; constant desmoplastic stroma; extensive infiltration of renal parenchyma; sometimes cytoplasmic mucin; sometimes carcinoma in situ in collecting ducts
Papillary RCC	Red brown tumor mass within kidney, no involvement of pelvic wall or lumen, often well circumscribed, usually cystic with areas of necrosis and hemorrhage	Usually low-grade tumor cell nuclei but may be high grade. Papillary structures with a single cell layer (*vs* multiple layers in the papillary structures of urothelial carcinoma), less often growth pattern including tubular, trabecular, or solid. Desmoplastic stroma not pronounced. Foamy macrophages frequent in the papillae of lower grade tumor

in all these three tumor types. Primary renal pelvic adenocarcinoma or metastatic adenocarcinoma may closely simulate collecting duct RCC, but they are rarely submitted to FS, since the former is exceptional whereas the latter is usually diagnosed by other means such as fine needle aspiration, and is not subjected to surgery.[6] Features that may facilitate these differential diagnoses are listed in Table 1.5 and Figs. 1.25–1.28.

FROZEN SECTION TO EVALUATE A CYSTIC RENAL MASS

Clinical Background

Up to 15% of renal tumor may be predominantly cystic. The Bosniak classification (Bosniak Class I–IV) is often used to classify renal cystic tumors on imaging. Class I tumors represent a unilocular mass with smooth and thin wall; Class IV tumors represent a multilocular mass with thick, shaggy wall and solid areas[27]; and Class II or III tumors are in between. The Class I tumor is thought to be benign and is usually not subjected to surgery. The Class II–IV tumors may histologically represent a large variety of lesions, including simple cyst with superimposing hemorrhage or infection, cystic nephroma, multilocular cystic RCC, and RCC with marked cystic changes secondary to necrosis or hemorrhage.[27,28] The treatment for these lesions is quite different and may depend on a specific diagnosis, which is usually not obtainable preoperatively, in spite of sophisticated renal imaging techniques or even fine needle aspiration.[28] FS is therefore may be requested before definitive treatment. Nevertheless, diagnostic failure of FS (often a false negative result) in this context has been often reported, reflecting sampling limitation or interpretational difficulty. These considerations limit the use of FS in the surgical treatment for cystic renal lesions.

Sometimes mass lesions develop in a kidney with diffuse cysts. The two most common conditions which cause bilateral diffuse renal cystic changes are *autosomal dominant polycystic kidney* and *acquired cystic kidney*, a condition associated with chronic dialysis. Symptomatic mass lesion including cyst infection, hematoma, or RCC may develop in these kidneys. Since the true nature of these masses may not be established by clinical or imaging findings, total nephrectomy may be needed and an intraoperative consultation may be requested.[29,30]

Specimen Handling

For a localized cystic renal mass, the submitted specimen may be a wedge biopsy of the cyst wall, the diagnosis of which may dictate a conservative approach for a benign lesion or radical resection for a malignant one. The entire specimen should be submitted for FS and, in case a diagnosis is not achieved, additional tissue should be requested.

Interpretation

The major differential diagnoses for a localized cystic mass include simple cyst, simple cyst with superimposing hemorrhage or infection, cystic nephroma, multilocular cystic RCC, RCC with marked cystic changes secondary to necrosis or hemorrhage, and mixed stromal and epithelial tumor.[28,31] Some features helpful for their differentiation are listed in Table 1.6. This table does not include cystic partially differentiated nephroblastoma which is also predominantly cystic, but is practically limited to the first two years of life.[31] These cystic lesions usually have distinctive gross features, which facilitate the differential diagnoses (Table 1.6 and Figs. 1.29–1.35). Some practical caveats pertinent to FS are emphasized. Identifying the epithelial cells lining the cyst wall is essential for a correct diagnosis. These cells, however, may be necrotic and replaced by inflammatory fibrous tissue as often seen in cystic papillary RCC (Fig. 1.35). Indeed, necrosis is an important clue for RCC and its presence should prompt an attempt to confirm this diagnosis. The presence of clear cells lining cyst wall, usually more than one layer, and/or clusters of clear cells within septa are required for diagnosing multilocular cystic RCC and differentiating it from other cystic tumors including cystic nephroma. During tissue preparation, these cells may be completely lost or appear only as mildly atypical bare nuclei reminiscent of lymphocytes, an artifact probably due to their delicate cytoplasm devoid of well-developed organelles or cytoskeleton (Figs. 1.31 and 1.32). In these situations, however, the highly vascularized and edematous stroma of the cyst wall or the septa, characteristic for clear cell RCC, is still present and, in our experience, is an important diagnostic clue (Figs. 1.31 and 1.32). The diagnostic pitfalls are highlighted by personally encountered cystic tumors diagnosed as "benign cyst" in FS since only fibrous wall is identified but, on permanent sections, show rare cyst lining cells characteristic for either clear or papillary RCC. These considerations imply a need for careful specimen sampling and for additional biopsies for FS if the subtle clues for RCC, as described above, are encountered in the initial FS slides (Figs. 1.29d and 1.35).

In the context of a mass lesion in a kidney with diffuse cystic changes, RCC is rare in autosomal dominant polycystic kidney and most renal masses in this condition represent intracystic hematoma or, less frequently, infection.[30] In contrast, RCC is very frequent and usually multifocal in acquired cystic kidney and, in about a third of cases, is associated with hemorrhage, which may be massive and mask the RCC.[29] Indeed, the presence of renal hematoma in the context of acquired cystic kidney should prompt a thorough search for RCC. In contrast, large hematoma may be "organized" at its periphery and appears as aggregations of atypical spindle cells, reminiscent of sarcomatoid RCC. The presence of admixed inflammatory cell including macrophages and hemosiderin granules may offer diagnostic clues.

TABLE 1.6 Differential diagnoses of cystic renal tumors.

	Gross	Lining epithelium	Septal stroma	Intraseptal epithelium
Simple cyst with infection or hemorrhage	*Unilocular*, usually in cortex, hemorrhagic, cheesy material in cyst wall or lumen	Flat or cuboidal non-clear cells in single layer; focal replacement of epithelium with fibrin, degenerated red blood cells, and fibroinflammatory tissue but NO necrosis	No septa	Not applicable
Cystic nephroma	Single *multilocular* mass, circumscribed or encapsulated, extension to perirenal or peripelvic soft tissue possible, smooth and thin wall molding to the cyst contour without solid mass, serous, gelatinous or serosanguinous cyst content, NO necrosis	Flat, cuboidal, or hobnail cells in single layer; rare clear cells (cyst lining cell may be focally clear, but this finding alone does not indicate renal cell carcinoma)	Vascularized fibrous tissue of variable celllularity; focal myxoid or myoid areas in some cases	Microcysts, complex branching tubules resembling renal tubules
Multilocular cystic RCC	Virtually identical to cystic nephroma	Almost always clear cells with low nuclear grade, in singe or multiple layers; focal loss of epithelium frequent	Fibrous and commonly calcified; focal myxoid and highly vascularized areas	Focal clusters of clear cells similar to cyst lining cells

| RCC with extensive cystic necrosis | *Multilocular* (usually clear cell RCC) or *unilocular*(usually papillary RCC) cyst due to necrosis and hemorrhage, solid tumor areas frequent | Cysts filled with hemorrhagic and necrotic debris, without tumor cell lining; cyst with mural nodules or microscopic clusters of clear or papillary RCC of variable nuclear grades | Thick, shaggy; myxoid and highly vascularized areas admixed with dense fibrotic areas | Tumor cells with necrosis and hemorrhage |
| Mixed stromal and epithelial renal tumor | Single *multilocular mass*, circumscribed but not encapsulated; frequent extension to peripelvic soft tissue, cysts always present but with different extent; some cases with pronounced solid areas and thick cyst wall | Cuboidal cells with focal intracystic papillary projection | Fibrous stroma with variable cellularity, thick-walled blood vessels, smooth muscle bundles | Microcysts, complex branching, tubules resembling renal tubules |

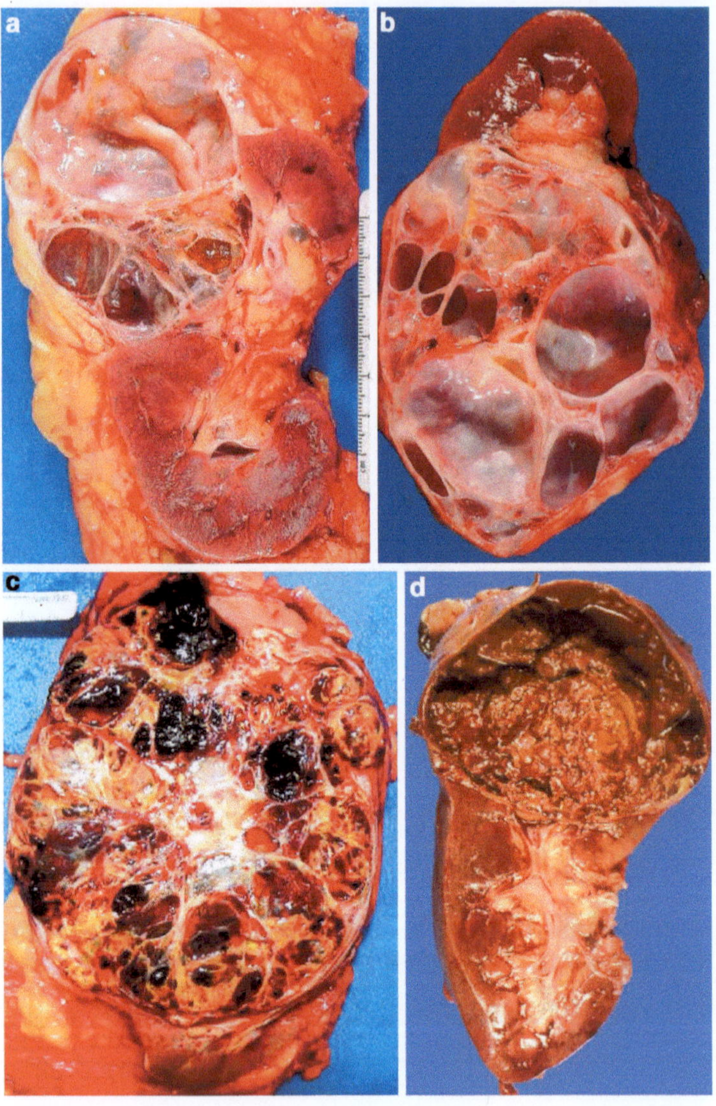

FIGURE 1.29 *Cystic renal neoplasm*. (**a**) *Cystic nephroma*: A single multi-locular, circumscribed mass composed of locules with smooth thin wall, without obvious necrosis or septal nodules. (**b**) Multilocular cystic clear cell RCC: Similar appearance as cystic nephroma. (**c**). *Clear cell RCC, with extensive cystic changes:* Cysts due to extensive necrosis and hemorrhage with multiple septal tumor nodules. (**d**) *Papillary RCC with cystic changes*: unilocular cystic tumor with necrosis of the wall.

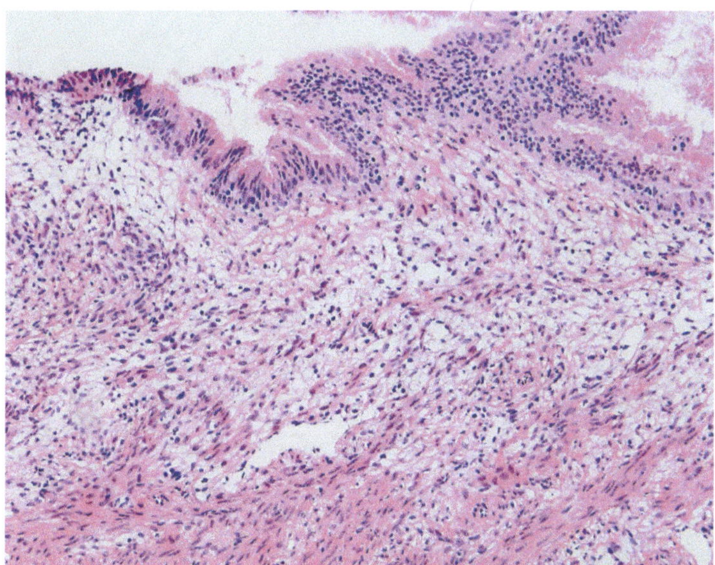

FIGURE 1.30 *Cystic nephroma*: The cyst is lined by cuboidal/columnar cells with intact eosinophilic cytoplasm. The stroma is fibromyxoid and vascular. Bundles of smooth muscle cells can be seen in both cystic nephroma and mixed stromal and epithelial tumor.

PARTIAL NEPHRECTOMY SPECIMENS

Clinical Background

Partial nephrectomy for renal tumors becomes more frequent due to increased detection of small and asymptomatic renal masses by imaging and the recently recognized importance of maintaining renal function for improving survival in patients with RCC maintaining renal function for long term-survival.[15] The later consideration is especially true for elderly patients, whose renal function may already be impaired by frequently associated conditions such as hypertension and diabetes. Its indications include (1) conditions where total nephrectomy renders the patient anephric.[32] These conditions include solitary kidney, bilateral synchronous RCC, genetic predisposition to multiple synchronous or sequential tumor as in von Hippel-Lindau (VHL) disease, hereditary papillary renal carcinoma syndrome, Birt-Hogg-Dube syndrome, and tuberous sclerosis; (2) small RCCs (usually <4 cm) confined to kidney, and (3) inflammatory masses or some benign renal tumors such as multilocular cystic nephroma, AML, and oncocytoma.[14]

Partial nephrectomy specimen is traditionally submitted for FS evaluation of *surgical margin* since complete tumor resection is

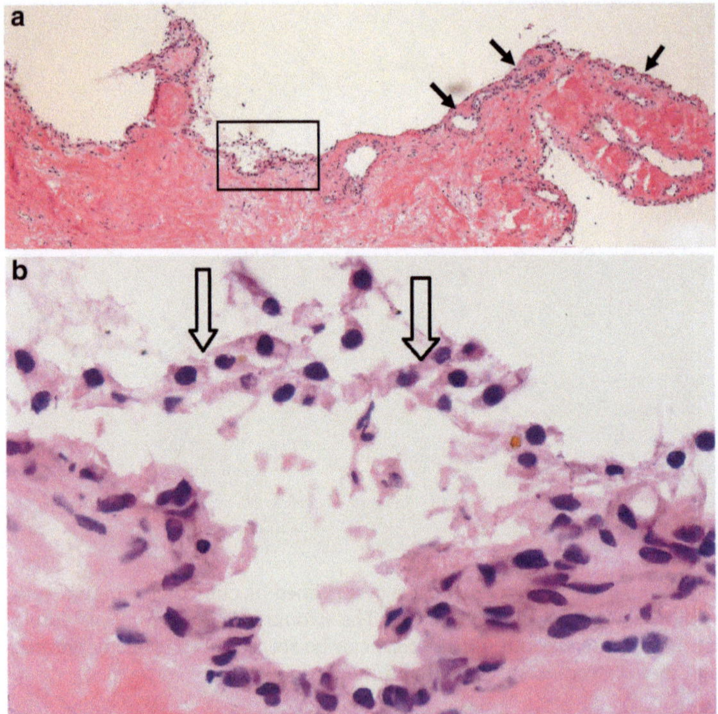

FIGURE 1.31 *Multilocular cystic RCC.* (**a**) A locule lined by fibrous stroma with superficial stromal vascularity (solid arrows) that can be recognized under low-power view, a characteristic feature, and a diagnostic clue. Most of the times, tumor cell lining is not obvious. (**b**) High-power view of the rectangle area in (**a**). The findings at low magnification should prompt careful examination and, in rare situation, inconspicuous tumor cells detached from the underlying wall can be found (*open arrows*). Touch prep usually yield a few bare small hyperchromatic nuclei, a characteristic feature of this tumor type (*see also* Fig. 1.6).

thought to be essential for successful treatment. However, refrain from routine FS consultation for surgical margin has been suggested by several more recent studies, citing rather frequent FS misinterpretation and more importantly, a lack of correlation of the surgical margin status with subsequent tumor recurrence, metastasis, or patients' survival.[33,34]

Partial nephrectomy can be performed by open surgery or laparoscopy. The implication of FS for surgical margin is somewhat different between these two approaches. This difference is

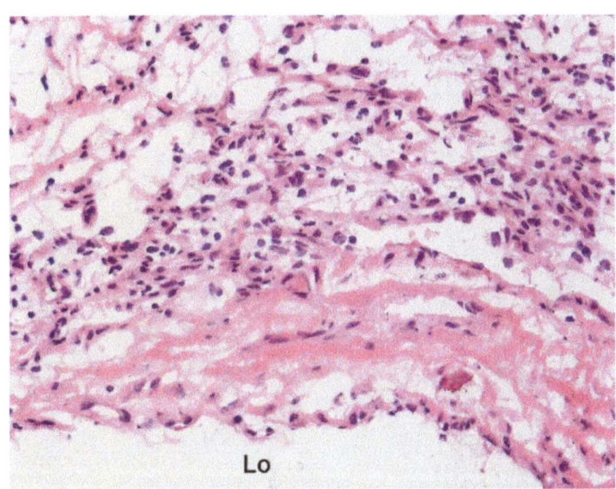

FIGURE 1.32 *Multilocular cystic RCC.* Septum of a locule (*Lo*) with vascularized stroma characterized by interconnecting thin-walled blood vessels lined by prominent endothelial cells set against an edematous background. Although there are no obvious tumor cells lining the locule or within the septum, this type of stroma is characteristic for multilocular cystic RCC. It presence should prompt further consideration for this diagnosis, including additional tissue sampling or request for more biopsies.

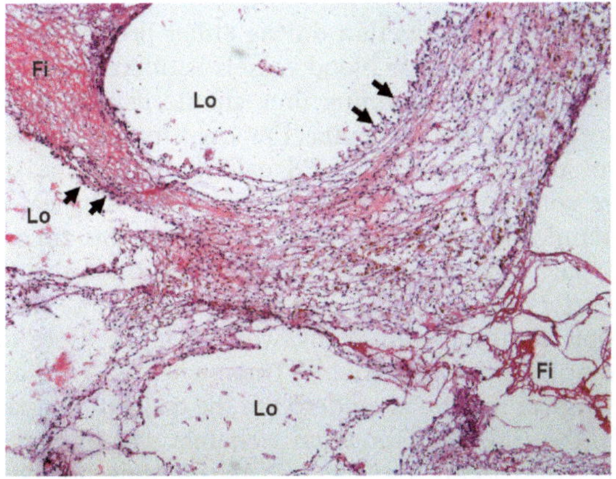

FIGURE 1.33 *RCC with extensive cystic necrosis.* The locules (*Lo*) are lined by tumor cells with clear cytoplasm (*solid arrows*). The same types of tumor cells may be present in the septa also, but these cells may be artifactually distorted with loss of the clear cytoplasm and may not be obvious. Hemorrhage and fibrin (*Fi*) are also noted within the septa or the lumens of the locules.

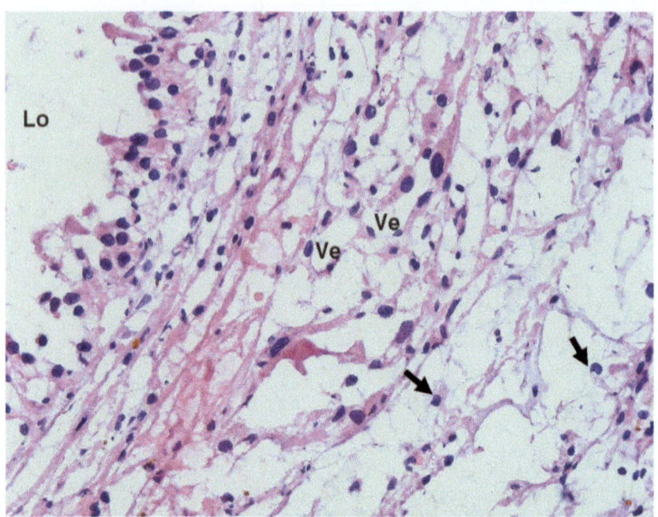

FIGURE 1.34 *RCC with extensive cystic necrosis*. Higher view of the Fig. 1.33. This locule (*Lo*) is lined by tumor cells with clear cytoplasm. The same type of tumor cells may be present in the septum also, but these cells may be artifactually distorted with loss of the clear cytoplasm and may not be obvious (*solid arrows*). Stromal thin-walled blood vessels with prominent endothelial cell lining are present (*Ve*).

related to the observation that during either procedure, the renal pedicle including the hilar blood vessels is often clamped to control bleeding, but the clamping time should usually be less than 30 min to avoid renal ischemia. For open partial nephrectomy, a positive surgical margin by FS calls for additional resection to achieve complete tumor resection with free surgical margins. This is technically possible in most cases since the time required for open partial nephrectomy is often less than the threshold for renal artery clamping. This scenario may not be the case for laparoscopic partial nephrectomy, which may be more time consuming that the open approach.[32] Thus, when an FS diagnosis of positive surgical margin is rendered in the context of laparoscopic approach, the threshold for renal ischemia was already reached and further excision of the surgical margin may not be feasible. The surgeon then can either complete the laparoscopic procedure regardless of the surgical margin status or proceed immediately to total nephrectomy.[32] Information on the tumor type provided by FS may influence this choice. Sometimes the surgical margin is evaluated not only by FS of the partial nephrectomy specimens but also by biopsy of the surgical bed.[35]

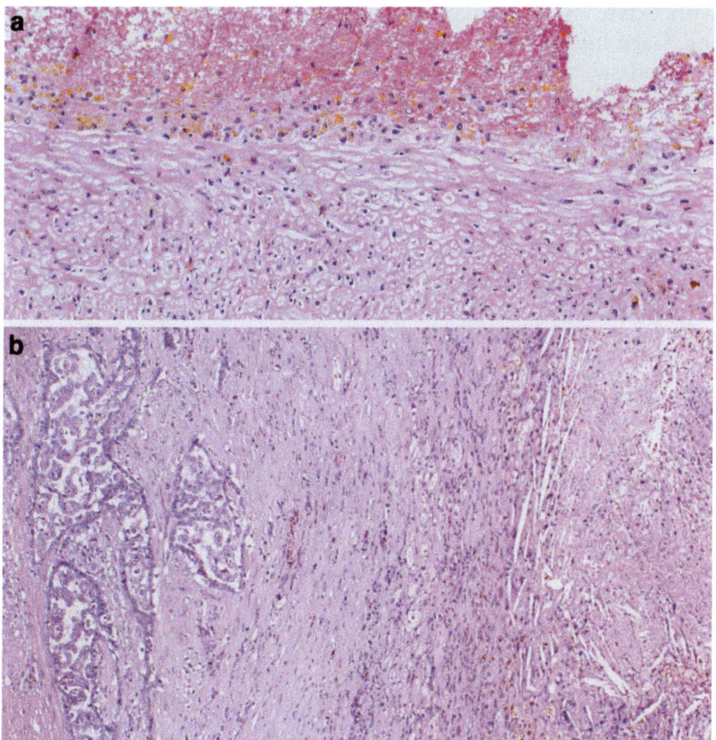

FIGURE 1.35 *Unilocular cystic papillary RCC.* (**a**) Most areas of the cystic tumor shown in Fig. 1.29d show necrotic material and macrophages lining a fibrous wall. These changes, however, strongly suggest the diagnosis of cystic papillary RCC. (**b**) Additional samplings for FS show an area of papillary carcinoma in the wall.

FS may be also requested for a *specific diagnosis* during partial nephrectomy, since tumor type may be one of the factors that determine whether partial nephrectomy is appropriate.[15] Furthermore, when the surgical margin is positive during laparoscopic partial nephrectomy, a specific diagnosis of a benign tumor such as AML or oncocytoma may negate the need for immediate total nephrectomy.[17,18]

Specimen Handling

Since partial nephrectomy is preferred for small peripheral and polar tumors, the resected specimen often includes renal tissue and perirenal adipose tissue. Central tumors, defined as those with extension to the collecting system or renal sinus by imaging,[36] are increasingly considered for partial nephrectomy. These resected specimens may also include renal sinus soft tissue and pyelocalyceal tissue, in addition to renal tissue and perirenal adipose tissue.[34,36]

Because of the complex anatomy of the kidney and the excretory system, the partial nephrectomy specimen is often disoriented or even disrupted, with the surgical margins difficult to identify. *In such case, orientation by the surgeon is essential.* The surgical margins may include perirenal soft tissue, renal parenchyma, pyelocalyceal tissue, and renal sinus soft tissue including blood vessels. Since RCCs chosen for partial nephrectomy are usually small (<4 cm) and remain confined to the kidney, the renal parenchymal margin is the most critical one, but other margins should also be evaluated.[34] The margins should be inked, followed by serial sectioning perpendicular to the renal parenchymal surgical margin to demonstrate the tumor and its relation to this margin.

Sometime, rather than submitting the partial nephrectomy specimen for evaluating surgical margin, biopsies of the remaining tumor bed after partial nephrectomy are separately submitted to evaluate surgical margin.[35] These biopsies are usually small and should be entirely submitted for FS. Misinterpretation is frequent in this situation (*see below*).[37]

Interpretation

Since the tumors selected for partial nephrectomy are usually circumscribed and even encapsulated, gross impression of a negative margin is usually accurate. However, Li et al. have shown that for clear cell or papillary RCC of 4 cm or less, microscopic extension of tumor tissue beyond the gross confine of the tumor can be seen in 19.5% of tumor at a distance of 0–5 mm (0.5 ± 1.3 mm).[38] These data speak against tumor enucleation and support the need for microscopic examination for the surgical margin. The minimum accepted surgical margin clearance has not been established.[34] Although a clearance of 1 cm was previously suggested, recent studies suggest that the size of the margin is not related to recurrence, and thus even a microscopic absence of tumor tissue at the inked surgical margin is adequate.[18,34] These observations are important since they facilitate the most essential goal of partial nephrectomy, that is maintaining as much functioning renal tissue as technically possible. Moreover, a large surgical margin clearance, for example 1 cm is evidently not possible for hilar/central tumors.[33,36] These complicated considerations withstanding, a positive surgical margin is indeed relatively rare (0–7.4%, mean 2.4%).[18,34]

Satellite tumor nodules may be encountered in up to 25% of all RCCs but in about 5–7% for those suitable for partial nephrectomy. In the latter instance, these nodules measure 0.1–2.8 cm and are situated 0.2–6.0 cm from the main RCC.[38,39] These data suggest that satellite nodules are not usually included in the partial nephrectomy specimens and are not a problem in FS.

Recognizing a free parenchymal surgical margin is usually straightforward when the partial nephrectomy specimen is submitted (Fig. 1.36). However, misinterpretation has been documented (Fig. 1.37), and this is rather often in case of small biopsy from the tumor bed.[37] Normal proximal renal tubules may closely simulate the tubular growth pattern in oncocytoma, a frequent tumor type in the context of partial nephrectomy (Fig. 1.38). Atrophic renal tubules often seen at the periphery of tumor may display enough structural distortion and reactive nuclear atypia, creating potential confusion with tumor tissue in FS (Fig. 1.39). Neoplastic tubules of low-grade RCC may look similar to benign renal tubules. The presence of glomeruli in tissue with misleading

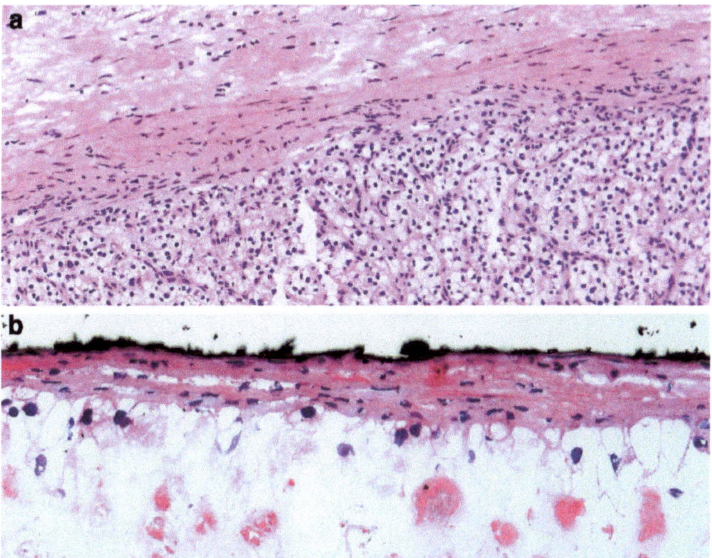

FIGURE 1.36 *Partial nephrectomy specimen*. (**a**) The tumor types selected for partial nephrectomy often are circumscribed or encapsulated, as seen in this low-grade clear cell RCC. (**b**) This observation supports the view that even a microscopic absence of tumor cells at the ink margin is acceptable as "free margin."

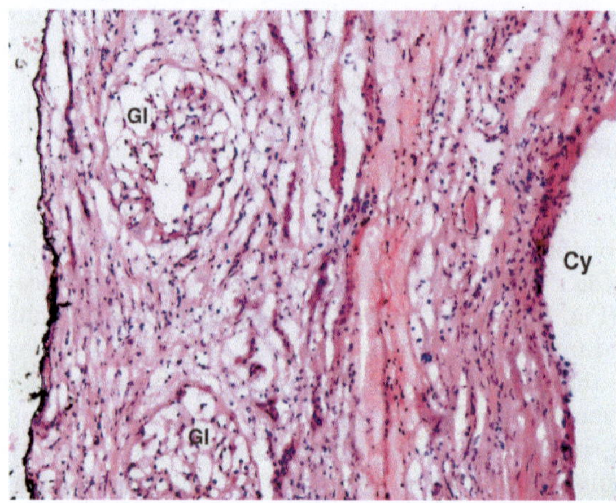

FIGURE 1.37 *Partial nephrectomy for a cystic clear cell RCC*. The tumor cyst (*Cy*) is not obviously lined by tumor cells. Whether tumor cells are present in the pericystic tissue is debatable, since, as mentioned previously, clear tumor cells in this context may be isolated and artifactually loose their clear cytoplasm, and are not readily identified. However, the presence of glomeruli (*Gl*) confidently indicates the absence of tumor tissue and thus a "free" surgical margin.

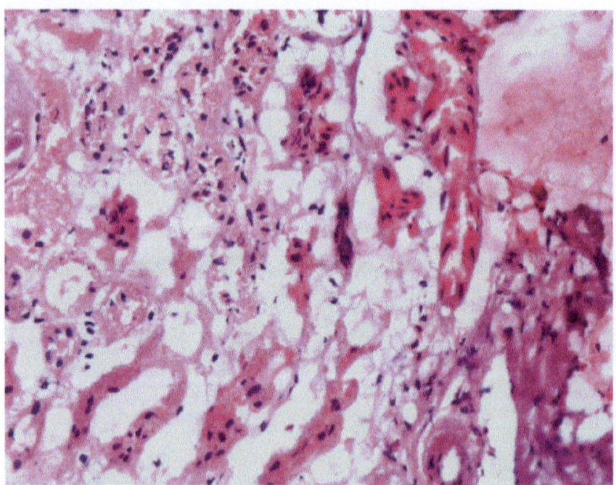

FIGURE 1.38 *Biopsy of the tumor bed during partial nephrectomy*. The submitted tissue is often distorted with artifactual changes. The proximal tubules may simulate oncocytoma. Identifying glomeruli admixed with these tubules confidently indicates the absence of tumor tissue. Even in case glomeruli are not obvious, the uniform tubular structures and nuclear regularity are compatible with proximal tubules (*see also* Figs. 1.18 and 1.20 for comparison with oncocytoma).

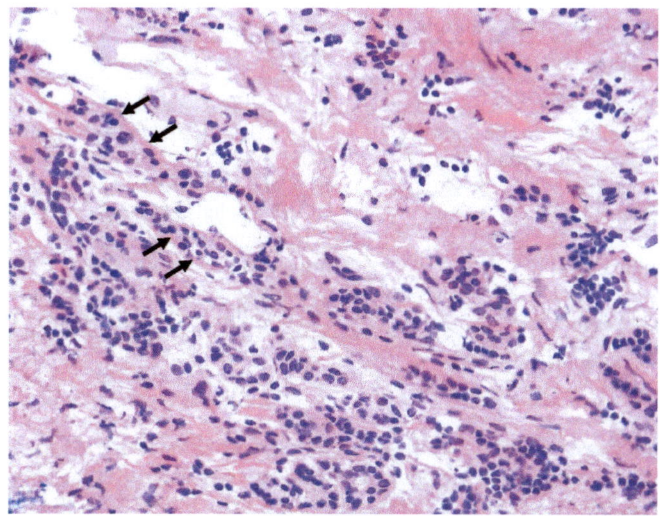

FIGURE 1.39 *Biopsy of the tumor bed during partial nephrectomy*. The peritumoral tissue may show tubular atrophy and interstitial fibrosis, simulating tumor tissue. A correct diagnosis should be facilitated by awareness of this type of changes, the uniform tubular appearance and thickened tubular basement membrane (*arrows*).

changes such as fibrosis or distorted tubules suggests the absence of tumor involvement (Fig. 1.37)

MULTIPLE RENAL MASSES AND EXTRARENAL MASSES

Clinical Background
FS may be requested for specific diagnoses when *multiple masses* are identified in one or both kidneys, or when *extrarenal masses*, including enlarged lymph nodes, are unexpectedly encountered during surgery for renal tumors.

Interpretation
Up to 10% of renal tumors are multiple or bilateral.[39] As listed in Table 1.7, these tumor masses may represent the *same* or *different* histological types.

Satellite Tumor Nodules in RCC
Up to 25% of sporadic RCCs show satellite tumor nodules of the same histological type as the main tumor, but the specific frequency depends on factors such as size, grade, or type of the index tumor.[40]

TABLE 1.7 Types of multiple renal masses.

Same histological types	Different histological types
Sporadic RCC	Clear cell RCC and angiomyolipoma
Clear cell RCC in the context of von Hippel-Lindau disease	Clear cell RCC and collecting duct RCC
Lymphoma	RCC and lymphoma
Angiomyolipoma	RCC, urthelial carcinoma, and lymphoma
Papillary RCC	Angiomyolipoma and cystic nephroma
Oncocytoma	Oncocytoma and chromophobe RCC

RCC = renal cell carcinoma

Since most of these satellite nodules are small and not obvious by renal imaging or during operation, they are not submitted to FS and are usually detected by permanent sections.

Multiple Renal Masses of the Same Histological Type

They may be encountered in the following situations: (1) multiple or bilateral AML seen in up to 70–85% of tuberous sclerosis patients,[19] (2) papillary RCC, which may be multifocal in up to 39% of cases,[41] and (3) oncocytoma, which may be multifocal in up to about 13% of cases.[11] Another condition that features mutifocal oncocytoma is renal oncocytosis, a recently described condition in which multiple oncocytomas, chromophobe RCCs, and tumors with hybrid features are found in the same kidney.[42] FS may be requested for these situations and awareness of them is the key to a correct diagnosis.

Multiple Renal Masses of Different Histological Types

They can be rarely seen in the same kidney, as listed in Table 1.7.[43,44] The gross and histological features of these lesions are similar to those of their respective isolated counterparts.

Renal Tumors in VHL Syndrome

Renal tumors develop in up to 70% of VHL patients during their life span. They display a morphological spectrum that includes variably sized, uni- or multilocular cysts, cysts with solid mural nodules, and solid tumors ranging from microscopic to unequivocal RCC.[45] They are almost always composed of clear cells of low-grade nuclei and simultaneously or sequentially present in the kidneys in various combinations, with RCC encountered in about 50% of patients at an age much younger than for sporadic RCC.[45]

These tumors are usually treated by conservative surgery including tumor enucleation and partial nephrectomy,[46,47] because (1) all of them are now known to be precursors of RCC, (2) new lesions continue to develop in both kidneys throughout life, which may require repeated surgery, and (3) this approach helps delay dialysis dependency until all renal tissue is removed. The renal lesions may be submitted to FS "to rule out RCC." It should be emphasized that all renal lesions in VHL patients have the same cytological features (being composed of clear cells with a low nuclear grade) and represent a morphological continuum within which the demarcation of RCC from the rest may be subjective and, indeed, has not been defined.[45] Since RCC metastasizes in 30–50% of VHL patients and this is the cause of death in 15–50% of them, *a more critical question with FS relevance is at what point RCC in this context can give rise to metastasis*.[45] In this aspect, Walther et al. noted that no patients with a solid tumor smaller than 3 cm left untreated for a median of 60 months developed metastasis.[46] These considerations should facilitate interpretation, when either a cystic or a solid renal tumor in a patient with VHL disease is submitted for FS.

Primary tumors of organs other than kidney often develop in VHL patients and, if encountered during renal surgery, must be differentiated from metastatic RCC. The most frequent problems in this context is *metastatic RCC* versus *pheochromocytoma* of the adrenal (Figs. 1.40 and 1.41), and *metastatic RCC* versus *a variety of primary cystic or solid pancreatic neoplasms*, all of which may feature a prominent clear cell component.[48]

Primary Renal Lymphoma

This tumor, defined as isolated renal involvement without systemic disease, is not rare. Six out of 200 renal tumors initially thought to be RCC were primary renal lymphoma.[49] Primary renal lymphoma may be identical to RCC on imaging studies, but up to a third of them may have unusual features, including multiple masses, predominantly perirenal plaque, or uni- or bilateral diffuse renal enlargement. In contrast, a renal mass in patients with systemic lymphoma may be RCC since a tenfold increase in the incidence of RCC is noted in these patients.[50] FS for a specific diagnosis may be requested since the treatment of choice for renal lymphoma is radiation/chemotherapy, whereas that for RCC is nephrectomy. The FS diagnosis of renal lymphoma is usually not problematic, even in a small biopsy, if the clinical context is aware of. The lesion is composed of compact lymphoid cells, which "crowd out" renal tissue and form nodules, or insinuate between intact renal tubules at the periphery of the nodules (Fig. 1.42).[49]

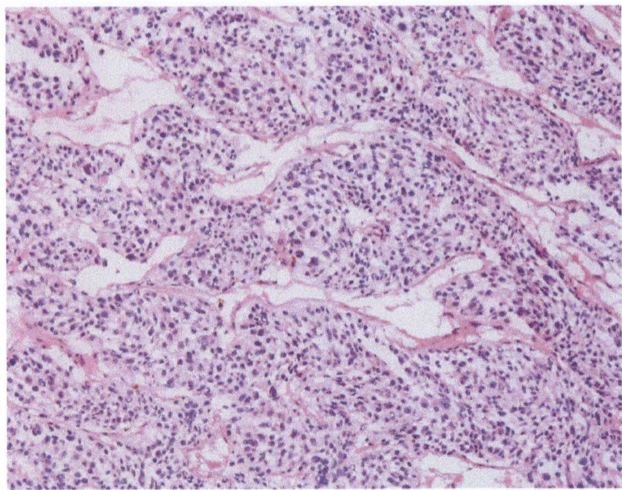

FIGURE 1.40 *Pheochromocytoma*. A large tumor involving both adrenal gland and kidney. Nests of tumor cells with abundant clear or faintly granular cytoplasm separated by dilated thin-walled blood vessels can simulate clear cell RCC.

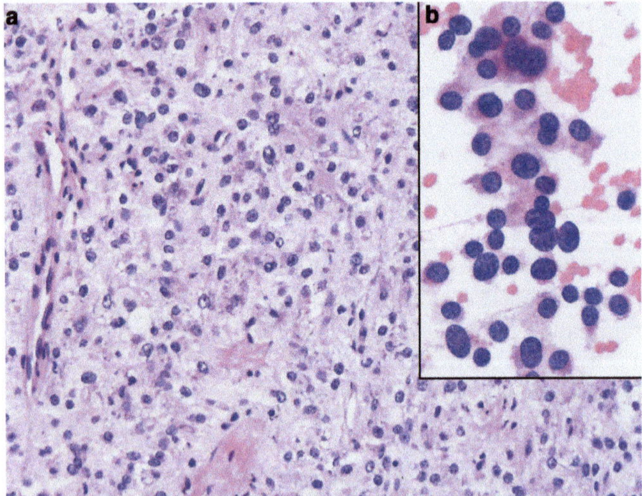

FIGURE 1.41 *Pheochromocytoma*. (**a**) Another area simulating clear cell RCC. (**b**) The touch prep, however, shows typical cytological features of pheochromocytoma, that is, small clusters and isolated cells or bare nuclei, with round nuclear contour and clumpy chromatin.

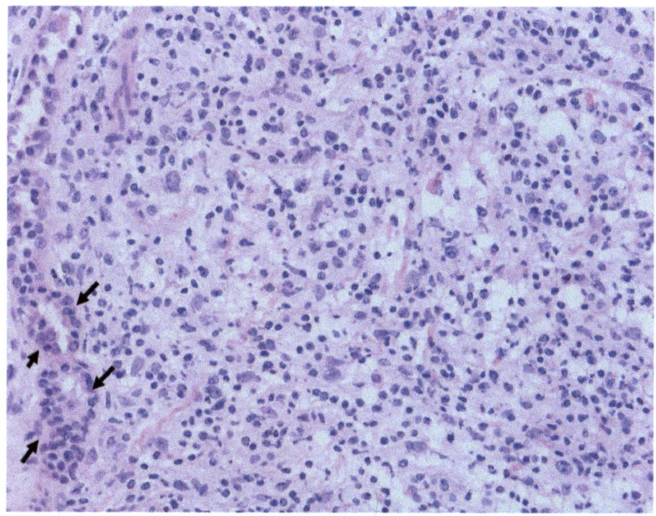

FIGURE 1.42 *Primary renal lymphoma.* Interstitial infiltration by lymphoid cells, several of which show atypical features, that is, large irregular nuclei and prominent nucleoli. Differentiation from interstitial inflammation is possible due to the presence of atypical lymphoid cells, and aggregation of the lymphoid cells to form gross or microscopic nodules, "crowding out" renal tubules (*arrows*).

Lymph Nodes

Nodal dissection is not routinely performed during total nephrectomy since this procedure does not improve survival, and clinically unsuspected nodal metastasis occurs in less than 5% of cases. Clinically recognized nodal metastasis often calls for nodal dissection for tumor staging and debulking purposes. Nodal metastasis is often suspected preoperatively by imaging, thus obviating the need for FS in most instances.[51] However, the enlarged lymph nodes may be due to *metastatic RCC, reactive lymphoid hyperplasia,* or *lymphoma.* Thus, FS may be requested. Ectopic adrenal cortex may appear as an isolated nodule in the hilar soft tissue, which may be confused with nodal metastasis on FS (Fig. 1.43).

Metastatic RCC often displays the same histological spectrum as the primary tumor; the primary tumor, however, may not be available for comparison since nodal FS may be performed prior to nephrectomy. Noting that nodal tumor tissue often show high-grade clear cell, papillary or sarcomatoid features may help with FS interpretation.[4] Micrometastasis may coexist with reactive lymphoid hyperplasia.

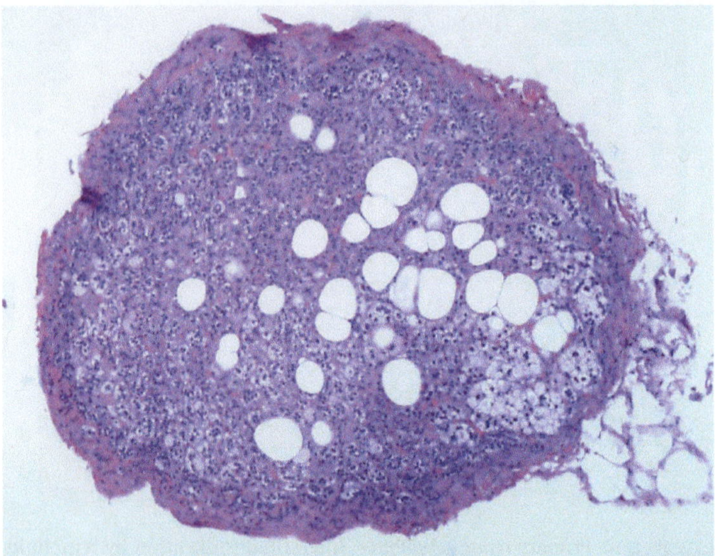

FIGURE 1.43 *Ectopic adrenal cortex* in permanent section. This nodule of ectopic adrenal cortex is detected in the nodal resection specimen for renal cell carcinoma. Other lymph nodes show reactive lymphoid hyperplasia. This type of lesion can simulate nodal metastasis of RCC in FS.

Since a tenfold increase in the incidence of RCC is recently reported in patients with lymphoma,[50] enlarged lymph nodes in the context of nephrectomy for RCC may be due to associated lymphoma. Awareness of this association aids in the differential diagnoses and ensures proper tissue triage for special studies, including flow cytometry and gene rearrangement. AML tissue may be encountered in lymph nodes but this represents multifocal tumor rather than metastasis.[19]

Extrarenal Masses

These masses may be encountered during surgery for a primary renal tumor and are often submitted for FS. These often include *adrenal masses* or *masses of other organs including peritoneum.*

Masses of other organs may be metastatic RCC or incidental lesions unrelated to RCC. In our experience, adrenal masses are most frequent and may include *RCC extending* or *metastatic to adrenal gland, adrenal cortical adenoma* or *nodule, adrenal cortical carcinoma extending to the kidney,* and *pheochromocytoma* (Figs. 1.40 and 1.41).

NEEDLE BIOPSY OF NATIVE OR TRANSPLANTED KIDNEYS

Clinical Background

These biopsies are usually "signed out" by a renal pathologist from specialized in-house units or referral laboratories. However, initial handling of these biopsies may require *immediate attention* of a general pathologist to determine whether the biopsy is adequate, so if additional tissue is needed, it can be obtained during the same procedure.

Specimen Handling

A spring-loaded biopsy device attached to a needle is currently used in most institutions. Although the needle can be of 14, 16, or 18 gauge, of which the smaller ones are usually preferred. Usually two or three tissue cores obtained by needle biopsy are submitted in saline or a preservative medium (usually a tissue culture fluid). How to divide these tissue cores for different studies is well described,[52] but is beyond the scope of this monograph. However, as mentioned above, requests may be made during the biopsy procedure to determine whether the biopsy is adequate.

Most native kidney biopsies are done for glomerular diseases. Many of the diseases accounting for renal allograft dysfunction are best represented in renal cortical tissue. *Therefore, the first goal of adequacy check is identifying renal cortical tissue including glomeruli.* Among various reported methods, we found the following accurate and technically feasible method, regardless of individual laboratory setting.[53] The tissue cores should be placed on a regular glass slide within a drop of preservative medium and examined under a regular light microscope.

Interpretation

The above procedure usually allows accurate identification of soft tissue (fat, skeletal muscle, fibrous tissue) and renal tissue including cortical tissue, glomeruli, larger blood vessels, and medullary tissue (Fig. 1.44). *Open* glomeruli are usually easily and accurately identified owing to the presence of red blood cells within the glomerular capillary lumens. Gently putting a glass coverslip on top of the cores will flatten them and enhance glomerular visualization. Sclerotic glomeruli or glomeruli with marked hypercellularity may not be visualized by this technique.

How much cortical tissue is considered adequate for a native kidney biopsy has not been established. The glomerular involvement in a specific renal disease may be patchy [segmental (a portion of the glomerular capillaries affected), global (all glomerular capillaries

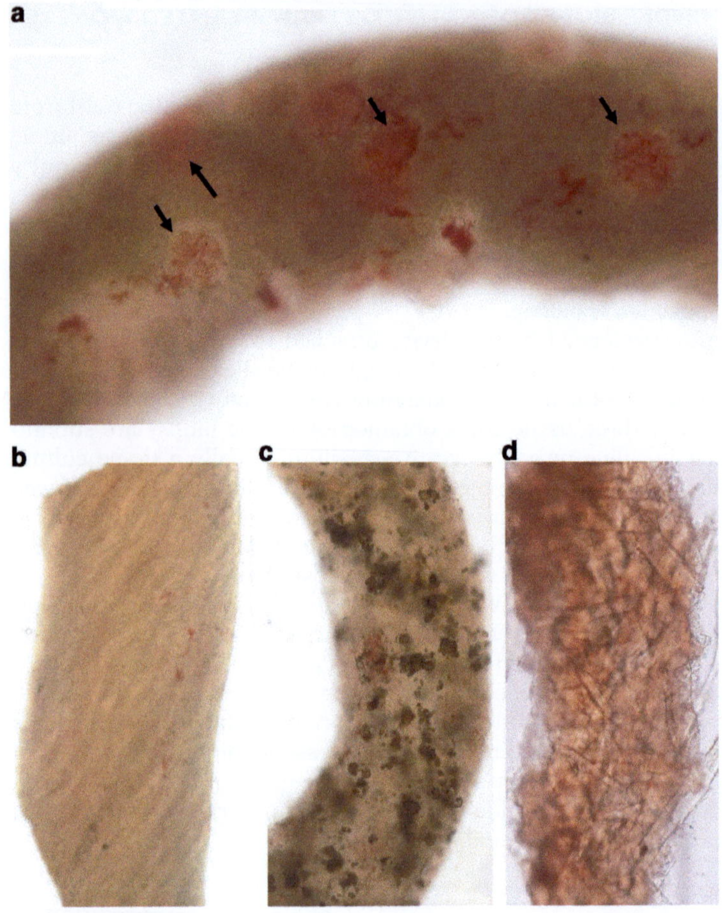

FIGURE 1.44 *Needle renal biopsy examined by regular light microscopy.* (**a**) Cortical tissue with several open glomeruli (arrows). (**b**) Medullary tissue characterized by a parallel distribution of renal tubules and an absence of glomeruli. (**c**) Cortical tissue with abundant crystalline deposition. The permanent sections show calcium oxalate nephropathy. (**d**) Skeletal muscle fibers.

of a glomerulus affected), focal (only some glomeruli affected), or diffuse (all glomeruli affected)]. Thus, a few glomerular capillaries are adequate for a global diffuse disease process, but a large number of them are needed for a focal segmental disease process. For example, for a disease process with an expected involvement of 10% of glomeruli, the chance to detect the lesion in a renal biopsy with ten glomeruli is 65%. This chance will increase to 95% for a disease process with an expected involvement of 35% of glomeruli.[54] These numbers, however, are derived from studies of tissue sections. How the number of glomeruli recognized by the above technique (three-dimensional) correlates with the number of glomeruli seen in the corresponding tissue sections (two dimensional) has not been determined, but the former is significantly higher in our experience. *We therefore empirically set the threshold for adequacy to include at least two cores of renal tissue with at least a half of the total tissue area being cortical tissue.*

For renal transplant biopsy, a retrospective study shows that the sensitivity for the diagnosis of rejection is 90% for one core and 99% for two cores.[55] The increasingly accepted Banff scheme for renal transplant biopsy stipulates that an adequate renal transplant biopsy should contain two tissue cores, with at least seven nonsclerotic glomeruli and two small artery profiles.[56] These numbers are intended for tissue sections. How to translate this threshold into immediate adequacy check of tissue cores is not clear. *We therefore empirically set the threshold for adequacy the same as for native kidney biopsy, that is, at least two cores of renal tissue with at least a half of the total tissue area being cortical tissue.*

DONORS' KIDNEYS

Clinical Background

Clinical criteria (no history of renal disease or hypertension, normal renal function, and normal urinalysis) are traditionally used to determine whether a donated kidney is accepted for transplantation. However, in response to the increasing shortage of donated kidney, kidneys from donors who do not meet these stringent criteria (expanded criteria donors) are *considered* for transplantation. *Biopsies from these kidneys with FS consultation* may play an important role in the clinical decision of whether these kidneys are accepted or rejected.[57] The possible indications for FS of a donated kidney are listed in Table 1.8. Morphological changes can be more sensitive than clinical parameters in predicting parenchymal injury and they may be pronounced even when renal function is normal.[58] This discrepancy usually encountered in kidneys from expanded criteria donors. These donors are often affected with conditions that may promote renal scarring and these conditions are best demonstrated by FS.[58] In USA, about 75% of the kidneys from these donors are biopsied, and about 41% of them were discarded, basing in part on the biopsy findings at FS.[57]

TABLE 1.8 Donors' kidneys: Reasons for frozen section consultation.

Conditions that may promote renal scarring
  Donors older than 60 years
  History of diabetes mellitus
  History of hypertension
  Cerebrovascular accident as the cause of death
Conditions that may promote renal necrosis
  Hypotension at time of renal harvesting
  Acute tubular necrosis
  Disseminated intravascular coagulation
  No heart beat at time of renal harvesting
Abnormal intraoperative observations
  Small kidney
  Granular renal surface
  Petechial renal hemorrhage
  Renal tumor
Abnormal laboratory findings during renal harvesting
  Serum creatinine greater than 1.5 mg/dl
  Hematuria
  Proteinuria
  Rapid deterioration of renal function

Specimen Handling

Either wedge or needle biopsy may be submitted. Wedge biopsy provides more tissue but may sample subcapsular cortical scars where globally sclerotic glomeruli may be overrepresented, a fact that should be taken in consideration during FS.[58] Needle biopsy may be more representative but may not provide enough tissue. In our practice, up to four pieces (less than 1 mm each) are obtained from the biopsies and saved for possible electron microscopy. The remaining tissue is divided into two portions and entirely submitted for FS. At the completion of FS, one block will be submitted for light microscopy and the other for immunofluorescent study. Permanent sections of the previously frozen tissue may show artifacts, which hamper precise interpretation. We, however, believe this limitation is well compensated for by the more accurate and timely available information if the entire specimen is submitted to FS. The exact definition for an adequate sampling has not been established. We empirically ask for cortical tissue with at least 25 glomeruli.[52,58] Additional tissue should be requested if this criteria is not met.

Interpretation

The following types of lesions should be sought: chronic parenchymal injury, intravascular coagulation, cortical necrosis, and glomerulonephritis.

TABLE 1.9 Grading of chronic renal injury in donors' kidneys.

Glomerulus
    Number of glomeruli in the biopsy
    Percentage of sclerotic glomeruli

Tubulointerstitium (percentage of cortical areas with tubular atrophy, interstitial fibrosis, and interstitial inflammation)

Normal	0–5%
Mild	6–25%
Moderate	26–50%

Blood vessels (fibrotic or hyaline intimal thickening of small arteries or arterioles as percentage of the original vascular lumen)

Normal-Mild	<25%
Moderate	26–50%
Severe	>50%

Evaluating *chronic parenchymal injury* should include separate evaluation of glomerular, tubulointerstitial, and vascular injury as listed in the Table 1.9. Although these parameters are separately evaluated, their severity roughly correlates with one another.[58] In FS, normal renal tissue may show tubular retraction associated with apparent expanded and edematous interstitium, which may be confused with chronic injury (Fig. 1.45). Chronic injury, however, should also include tubular atrophy, fibrous stroma, and increased stromal cellularity including inflammatory cells (Fig. 1.46). As mentioned above, subcapsular scar should be ignored in evaluating the extent of chronic tubulointerstitial injury (Fig. 1.47). Sclerotic glomeruli may be difficult to identify in FS and a longer exposure to eosin may be helpful (Figs. 1.47 and 1.48). The vascular changes most often include arteriolar hyalinosis and arterial fibrointimal thickening (Table 1.9 and Figs. 1.49 and 1.50) *The morphological threshold of chronic injury for accepting or rejecting a donor's kidney has not been established.*[58,59] We therefore accurately report the observed changes together with their respective severity, so that the transplant surgeon can incorporate them in their preferred final decision scheme. For example, one group declines to transplant the donated kidney when significant injury (defined as more than 20% glomeruli with global sclerosis or more than mild tubulointerstitial or vascular injury) is noted in any compartment.[58,60]

Intravascular coagulation may be seen in up to 10% of unselected donor renal biopsies and this incidence may be as high as 30% in those who died of brain trauma (probably due to sudden

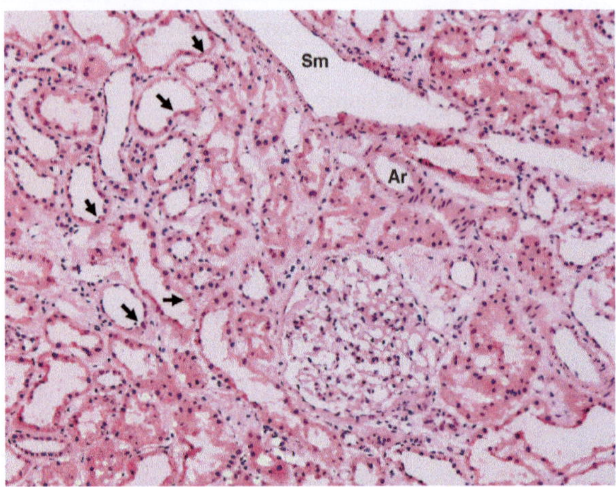

FIGURE 1.45 *Donor kidney*. No pathological alteration. The tubules are not "back-to-back" but are separated by a widened interstitial space: This is an almost constant artifactual change. The tubules have normal sizes and shapes. There is focal flattening of the tubular epithelial cells (*solid arrows*), which may represent artifact or acute tubular cell injury, but should not affect the decision to accept or deny the donor kidney. The small artery (*Sm*) and arteriole (*Ar*) are normal with an inconspicuous intima.

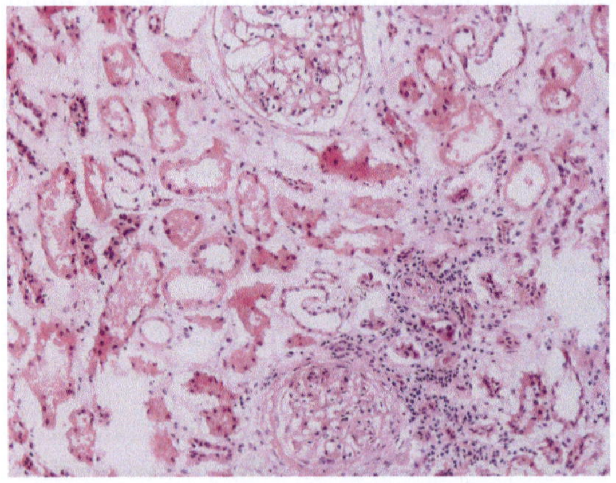

FIGURE 1.46 *Donor kidney*. Focal chronic tubulointerstitial injury (lower right) characterized by tubular trophy, thickened tubular basement membrane, interstitial fibrosis, and mild interstitial inflammation. A glomerulus in this area also shows features of chronic ischemic injury, including reduced size, mesangial sclerosis, and thickened glomerular capillaries. These changes contrast with the adjacent normal kidney tissue.

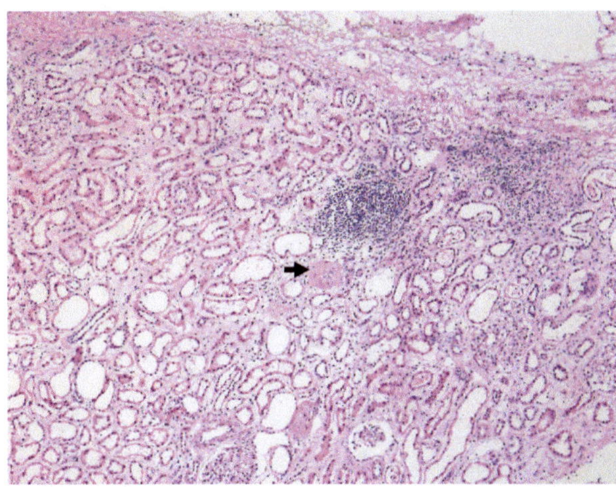

F IGURE 1.47   *Donor kidney*. A subcapsular scar characterized by a triangular area of chronic tubulointerstitial injury and sclerotic glomeruli (*arrow*) just below the renal capsule. The kidney tissue elsewhere is unremarkable. Area like this should be ignored in evaluating the extent of chronic tubulointerstitial injury.

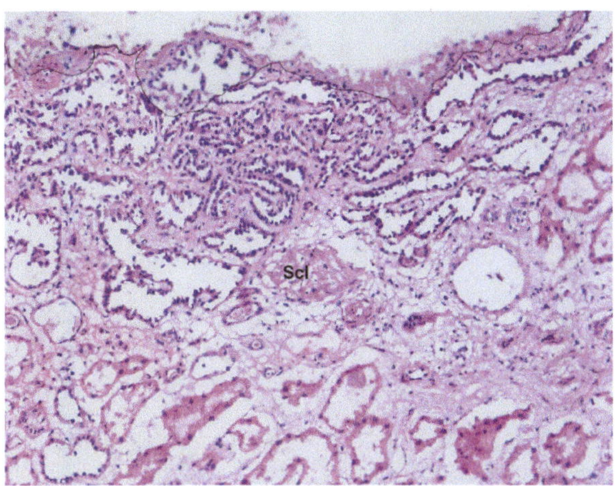

F IGURE 1.48   *Donor kidney*. A subcapsular microscopic papillary adenoma. Although this type of lesion is often associated with chronic ischemic renal injury, it should not by itself preclude donor acceptance. Adjacent to the adenoma is an area of chronic tubulointerstitial injury including a sclerotic glomerulus (*Scl*).

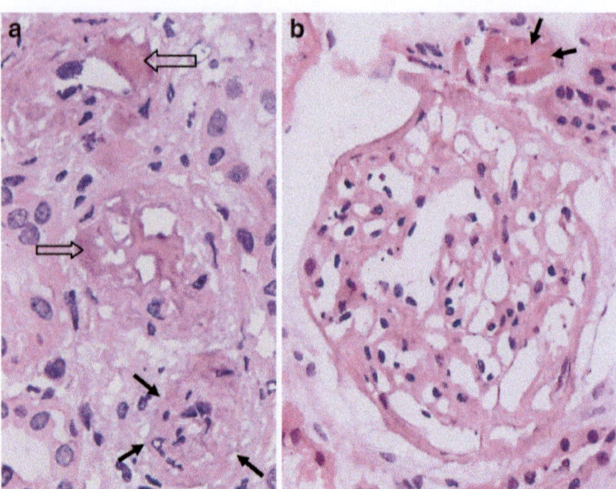

FIGURE 1.49 *Donor kidney.* (**a**) An arteriolar profile with marked intimal fibrous thickening and almost complete obliteration of the vascular lumen (*solid arrows*). Two arteriolar profiles with segmental hyalinosis (*open arrows*), intimal fibrous thickening, and almost complete obliteration of the vascular lumen. (**b**) Circumferential arteriolar hyalinosis with almost obliteration of the vascular lumen (*arrows*).

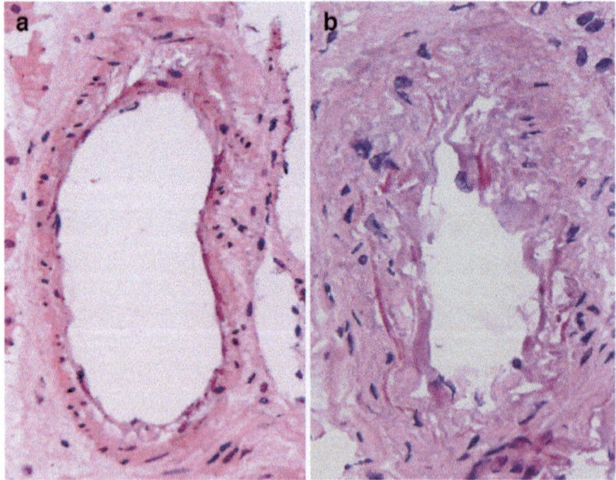

FIGURE 1.50 *Donor kidney.* (**a**) Normal small artery, with well-defined but thinned media and inconspicuous intima. (**b**) A small artery with thickened wall including intimal fibrosis, encroaching probably more than 50% of the original vascular luminal area.

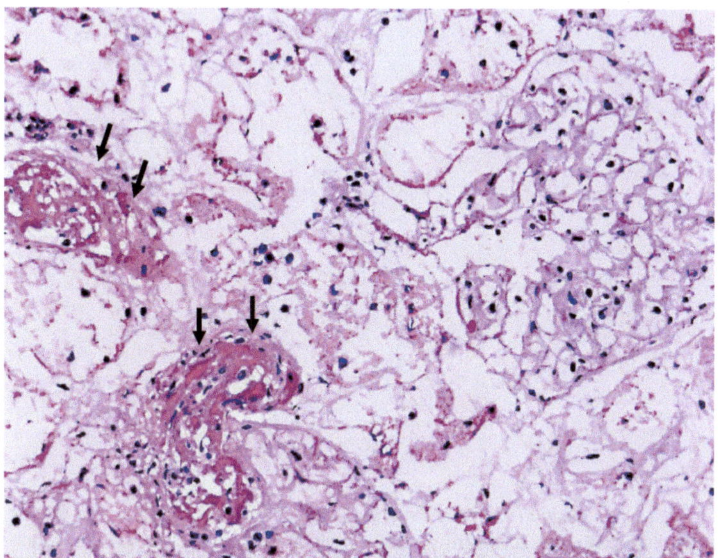

FIGURE 1.51 *Donor kidney*: Intravascular coagulation (*arrows*) with cortical necrosis characterized by necrosis of all tissue components including tubules and glomeruli.

release of brain thromboplastin, a potent procoagulant, into the circulation).[61] This is a frequent cause of petechial hemorrhage observed on the renal surface intraoperatively. It is characterized by the presence of fibrin thrombi in rare or many glomerular capillaries and in other blood vessels much less frequently. These thrombi, once being aware of, should be easily detectable in FS (Fig. 1.51). Intravascular coagulation, even when severe, should not, by itself, be a contraindication for transplantation, since the long-term outcome of the transplanted kidneys with this lesion is comparable with controls.[61] However, severe and prolonged intravascular coagulation may induce cortical necrosis which renders the kidney unacceptable.

Cortical necrosis is characterized by necrosis of all cortical elements including *tubules and glomeruli* and the injury is irreversible. Cortical necrosis in donor kidney is very rare and almost always due to massive intravascular coagulation.[61] Cortical necrosis must be differentiated from acute tubular cell injury, in which acute injury, including necrosis, is limited to the tubular cells and

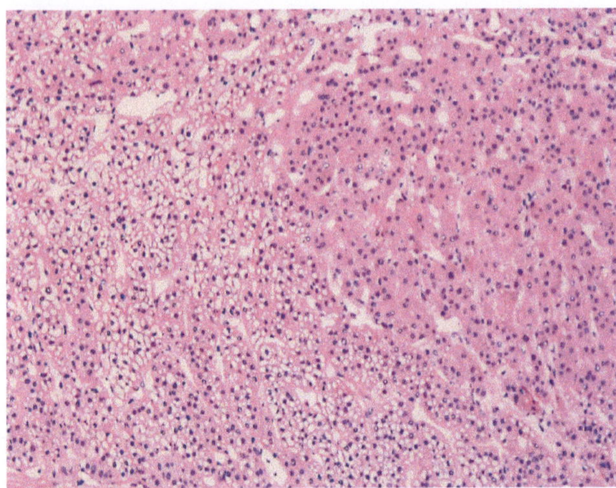

FIGURE 1.52 *Adrenal cortical heterotopia* can be seen within the donor kidney and must be differentiated from renal cell carcinoma. The presence of both clear and granular cell types and a uniform trabecular pattern are diagnostic clues.

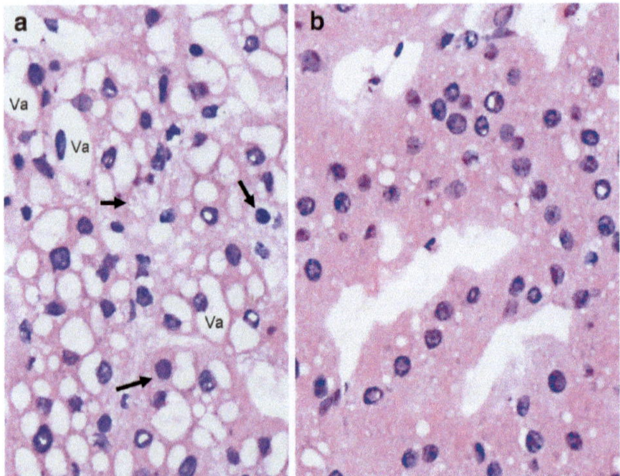

FIGURE 1.53 *Adrenal cortical heterotopia.* (**a**) At higher magnification, the cells in the clear area may show a single cytoplasmic vacuole (*Va*), an artifact; but may display finely vacuolated cytoplasm (*arrows*), typical for the adrenal cortical cells in the zona fasciculata or zona glomerulosa. (**b**) The cells with granular cytoplasm display uniform round nuclei and a trabecular growth pattern typical for the cells in the zona reticularis.

the injury is potentially reversible. Recognizing cortical necrosis in FS may not be difficult, especially in case of frank coagulative necrosis or infarct (Fig. 1.51), but acute tubular injury may be very difficult to diagnose since many changes characteristic for acute tubular injury are either masked by FS or confused with FS artifacts (Fig. 1.45). Fortunately, acute tubular injury is not a reason for rejecting a kidney since, when transplanted, such kidney may have delayed graft function but enjoys a normal long-term outcome.[58]

Donors with a significant *glomerulonephritis* are often recognized and eliminated by clinical criteria. Mild glomerulonephritis, which is often asymptomatic, may escape FS detection only to be diagnosed on permanent studies. This sequence is probably most frequent for IgA nephropathy, a disease with very high prevalence in some ethnic groups. Other diseases have been rarely reported including lupus nephritis, membranous glomerulonephritis, and membranoproliferative glomerulonephritis.[62] Fortunately, these mild forms of donor-transmitted glomerulonephritis have not shown to adversely affect the long-term graft and may even regress.[58]

Grossly visible *subcapsular nodules* may be identified during renal harvesting. They are usually excised and submitted for FS for both diagnosis and surgical margin. An accurate diagnosis is important in this context. If a benign tumor such as cyst, leiomyoma, AML, papillary adenoma (papillary growth, low nuclear grade, less than 0.5 cm), or adrenal cortical heterotopia is identified, it should not be a cause for rejecting the kidney.[58] True RCC that escapes clinical screening are, however, identified in up to 0.3% of donated kidneys.[63] Whether it precludes transplantation has not been determined but probably depends on many features including tumor size, histological type, and nuclear grade. FS should be helpful in this context. A misdiagnosis of RCC for adrenal cortical heterotopia may result in the discard of not only the kidney with the lesion but also the contralateral kidney. This happens in 3 of the 12 renal cortical nodules reported by Ditonno et al.[64] Conversely, transplantation of a kidney in which RCC is incorrectly diagnosed as adrenal cortical heterotopia by FS may result in subsequent graft nephrectomy.[64] A surgical margin negative for tumor is also important since a positive margin may be associated with subsequent metastasis.[65] Among the RCC types, adrenal cortical heterotopia may closely simulate a low-grade clear cell RCC. Features that facilitate their differential diagnoses are illustrated in Figs. 1.52 and 1.53.

Chapter 2
Urinary Bladder, Ureter, and Urethra

Steven S. Shen, Jae Y. Ro, Seth P. Lerner,
andL uan D. Truong

REASONSF ORINT RAOPERATIVE PATHOLOGYCO NSULTATION

Intraoperative pathology consultation for urinary bladder specimens is relatively infrequent, accounting for less than 5% of all frozen sections (FS) diagnosis requests in previous studies.[1,66,67] Wide use of transurethral cystoscopy allows preoperative biopsy or resection of most bladder lesions for histological diagnosis. However, intraoperative pathology consultation remains essential for guidance of surgery in several selective instances. The reasons, diagnostic usefulness, and pitfalls of FS of urinary bladder, ureter, and urethra specimens will be discussed.

There are number of reasons for FS and they are related to the types of specimen submitted to pathology laboratory. These indications vary among different hospitals and different surgeons. The types of specimen submitted for FS may include:

1. Evaluation of surgical margin status including ureteral, urethral, and soft tissue margins during radical cystectomy for bladder urothelial carcinoma
2. Evaluation of bladder mucosal and parenchymal resection margin in partial cystectomy specimen
3. Intraoperative diagnosis of transurethral biopsy or resection of bladder lesions
4. Intraoperative diagnosis of extravesical or bladder peritoneal nodules or masses
5. Evaluation of pelvic lymph nodes for metastatic urothelial carcinoma
6. Bladder neck margin during radical prostatectomy for prostate adenocarcinoma

L.D. Truong et al., *Frozen Section Library: Genitourinary Tract,*
Frozen Section Library 2, DOI 10.1007/978-1-4419-0691-5_2,
© Springer Science+Business Media, LLC 2009

TABLE 2.1 Reasons for intraoperative consultation in 162 consecutive urinary bladder specimens (materials from The Methodist Hospital, Houston, TX).

Gross consultation	4%
The presence and extent of a lesion in radical cystectomy specimen	
Frozen section consultation	96%
Status of ureteral margins for radical cystectomy	55%
Status of other margins (urethra, soft tissue) for radical cystectomy	10%
Margins of partial cystectomy	2%
Diagnosis of bladder tumor	4%
Diagnosis of bladder tumor with extravesical extension	2%
Pelvic nodal dissection	19%
Status of bladder neck margin for radical prostatectomy for prostate cancer	3%
Others (during cystectomy)	1%

A list of reasons and relative frequency for intraoperative pathological consultation from 162 consecutive bladder specimens from one institution is shown in Table 2.1. The three most frequent requests were for evaluation of ureteral margin during radical cystectomy, pelvic lymph node metastasis, and evaluation of urethral and extravesical soft tissue margins.

EVALUATION OF THE SURGICAL MARGINS DURING RADICAL CYSTECTOMY OR CYSTOPROSTATECTOMY

Clinical Background

Cystectomy with pelvic lymph node dissection is the standard therapy for muscle invasive bladder carcinoma and is sometimes indicated for high-grade nonmuscle invasive urothelial carcinoma that is resistant to conventional intravesical therapy or tumors with adverse prognostic features, such as extensive lymphovascular invasion or aggressive histological variants, such as micropapillary urothelial carcinoma. During radical cystectomy or cystoprostatectomy, the most frequent FS request is evaluation of ureteral, urethral, and perivesical soft tissue margins. It is well known that urothelial neoplasia is frequently multifocal and may involve the mucosal resection margins including ureteral and urethral mucosal margins, in the form of urothelial carcinoma in situ or pagetoid mucosal spread of adjacent urothelial carcinoma (pagetoid in situ carcinoma) or rarely separate foci of invasive carcinoma.

Ureteral Margin

Although the effectiveness of routine FS of ureteral margin is brought into question in a number of studies,[68-70]achieving a negative ureteral margin when feasible is desirable for urinary diversion in order to reduce the risk of recurrence at the ureterointestinal anastamosis. In a number of previous studies, the incidence of high-grade dysplasia/carcinoma in situ of the ureteral margins ranges from 4.8% to 9%.[69-71] In most hospitals including ours, bilateral distal ureteral margins are routinely submitted for FS; if the margin is positive for high-grade dysplasia/carcinoma in situ, additional ureteral tissue with new margin might be taken if clinically appropriate.

Urethral Margin

FS of distal prostatic urethra is requested to ensure that no high-grade dysplasia/carcinoma in situ is present at the urethral margin before performing continent urinary diversion with construction of an orthotopic neobladder.[72]

Perivesical Soft Tissue Margin

In situations when clinical examination and surgical findings are equivocal, FS might be requested to determine the resectability or adequacy of tumor resection.

Specimen Handling

The goal of FS of ureter and urethra is to evaluate the mucosal margin for high-grade dysplastic changes, carcinoma in situ, or invasive carcinoma. The first thing to do is to identify the lumen of the specimen by using a probe and embed the entire specimen with the lumen parallel to the cutting surface. For longer segment of ureter, the true margin is usually designated by the surgeon. If orientation is not provided, clarification with the surgical team might be necessary. The soft tissue margins may be separately submitted as small biopsy before cystectomy. For cystectomy specimen, this margin of concern is usually designated by the surgeon using suture or ink.

Interpretation

For the ureteral or urethral margin, any invasive tumor or high-grade dysplasia/carcinoma in situ would reflect a positive margin. In most cases, the interpretation is straightforward. The diagnoses may be divided into three broad categories: nondysplastic, atypia but not further classified, high-grade dysplasia/carcinoma in situ or invasive carcinoma. For a well-oriented and well-prepared cross section, normal ureter has a stellate lumen with loose subepithelial connective tissue surrounded by muscularis propria (Figs. 2.1–2.4). The diagnosis of low-grade dysplasia should be avoided if possible because of the poor diagnostic reproducibility and lack of standard treatment options (Figs. 2.5 and 2.6). The most useful diagnostic criteria for high-grade dysplasia/CIS include architectural changes including loss of polarity, nuclear crowding, and overlapping and nuclear abnormalities including nuclear enlargement, hyperchromasia, pleomorphism, and increased mitoses with or without abnormal mitoses (Figs. 2.7–2.14). According to the most recent classification of urothelial neoplasms by the World Health Organization/International Society of Urologic Pathology (WHO/ISUP), not only full thickness involvement but also partial involvement of the urothelium by cells with hyperchromatic, enlarged, and irregular nuclei is qualified for the diagnosis of high-grade dysplasia/carcinoma in situ. In our experience, a positive margin for high-grade dysplasia/carcinoma in situ or invasive carcinoma

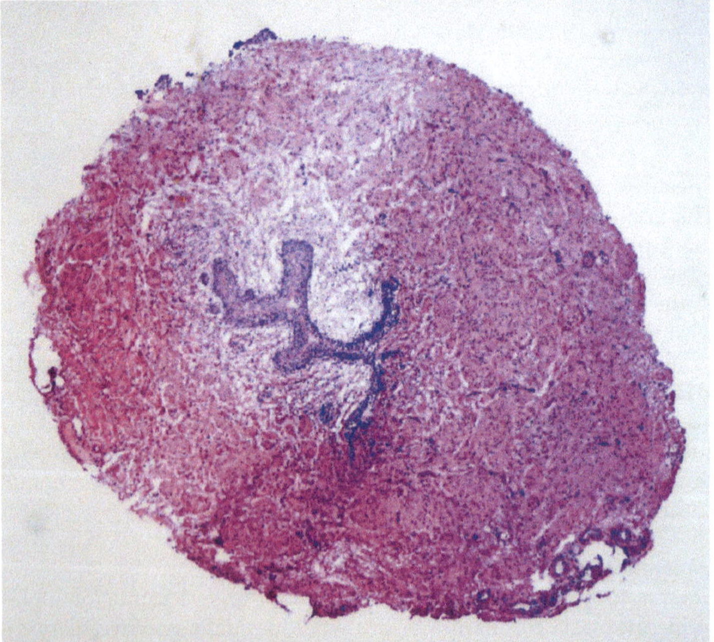

FIGURE 2.1 *Normal ureter*. Well-orientated cross section of the ureter is critical for accurate frozen section evaluation of urothelium. Multiple levels might be necessary to see the entire profile of the urothelium.

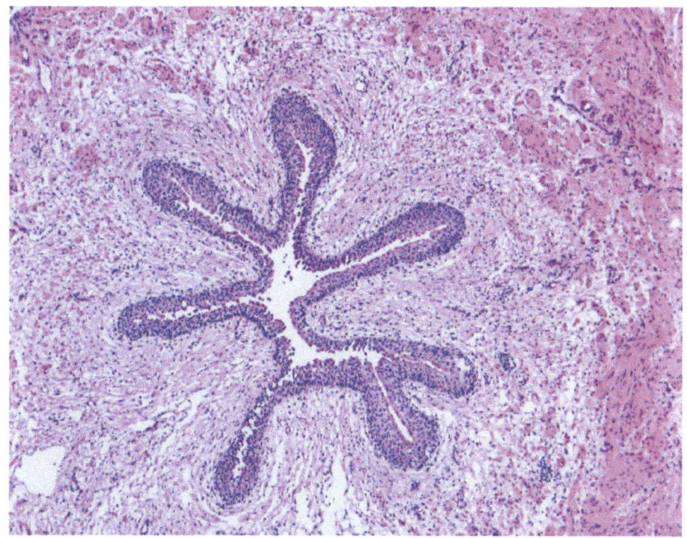

FIGURE 2.2 *Normal ureter.* Stellate-shaped lumen covered by urothelium of variable thickness. The subepithelial tissue is composed of loose fibroconnective tissue with thin-walled vessels and minimal chronic inflammatory cells. The muscularis consists of tightly packed smooth muscle bundles.

usually shows diffuse involvement of the urothelium by neoplastic cells. Sometimes, the segment of the ureter with high-grade dysplasia/carcinoma in situ shows dilation, chronic inflammation, and complete or partial sloughing of the neoplastic urothelial cells (Fig. 2.7). These changes are frequently associated with increased vascularity and inflammation in the subepithelial connective tissue. Increased vascularity and inflammation in the lamina propria with sloughing of the surface urothelium in FS should raise the possibility of high-grade dysplasia/carcinoma in situ and prompt examination of deeper tissue levels, or recommendation for new surgical margin if possible.

Diagnostic pitfalls include significant inflammation resulted from prior therapy, catheterization, or infection. Reactive atypia is a frequent finding and is often associated with inflammation, edema, or fibrosis of lamina propria. Be aware that urothelial cell nuclei in FS are often artifactually enlarged and mildly hyperchromatic due to freezing and cutting artifact, that is they seem more atypical than their counterparts in permanent sections. The chromatin of reactive urothelial cells is paler and evenly distributed. There is uniform nuclear enlargement and often small nucleoli.

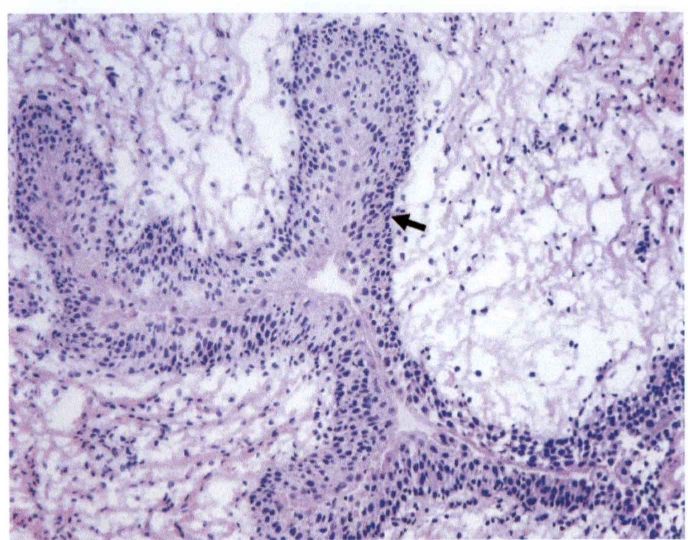

FIGURE 2.3 *Normal ureter.* The urothelial lining of ureter is composed of urothelial cells with variable thickness ranging from two to six cells with intact umbrella cells on the surface. The subepithelial connective tissue is composed of loose fibroconnective tissue with variable edema. There is a sharp demarcation of urothelial lining from the subepithelial tissue by a thin layer of basement membrane (*arrow*).

The cell polarity is maintained, and intraepithelial inflammatory cells are often present (Figs. 2.15–2.17).

En face section of the distal urethral surgical margin including urethra and periurethral soft tissue is often acceptable for evaluation of urethral margin status. Because of the retraction of the urethra, multiple levels might be necessary to show the urothelium for evaluating the mucosal margin. The key is to recognize the complexity of histological components in this location. In many patients, the urethral mucosa can be denuded due to intravesical therapy or intubation; special attention should be paid to evaluate periurethral glands or ducts for any dysplastic changes. Pagetoid spread with a few high-grade malignant cells is sufficient for the diagnosis of urothelial carcinoma in situ. Positive urethral margin is a very uncommon finding. The diagnosis of high-grade dysplasia/CIS and its pitfalls are similar to that of FS of the ureter (Figs. 2.18–2.20).

Invasive urothelial carcinoma on the ureteral or urethral margins is a rare finding during intraoperative FS evaluation, with an

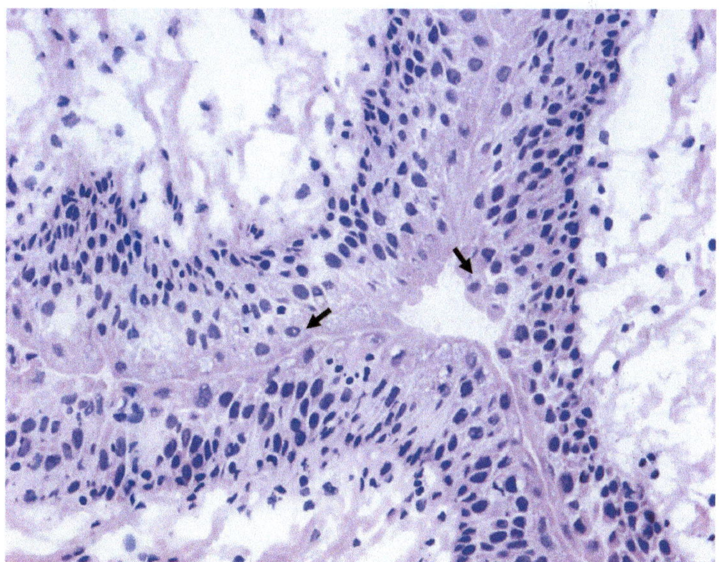

FIGURE 2.4 *Normal ureter*. High-power view showing intact umbrella cells, with abundant eosinophilic and vacuolated cystoplasm (*arrow*) lining on the surface of the urothelium. The urothelial cells are all perpendicular to the basement membrane. The cells, in general, are relatively uniform, ovoid, or elongated. The basal cells are often smaller and have a high N/C ratio. On frozen section, because of freezing and cutting artifact, the cells often show mild loss of polarity and mild variation of nuclear sizes.

incidence of 0.2% in one study. It is most often associated with mucosal carcinoma in situ (Figs. 2.21–2.23). Of note, in poorly differentiated carcinoma or rare variants of urothelial carcinoma, such as micropapillary, plasmacytoid, or signet ring cell carcinoma, isolated or small clusters of tumor cells can be seen in the periureteral soft tissue at the surgical margin, without involvement of the urothelium.

The interpretation of perivesical soft tissue margins is usually straightforward. Invasive urothelial carcinoma at the margin is characterized by often highly atypical tumor cells in nests or single cells and surrounded by desmoplasia (Figs. 2.24 and 2.25). Cautery artifact and chronic inflammation can be problematic. Peritoneal fat necrosis with fibrosis is also not an uncommon finding. Occasionally reactive endothelial cells can simulate invasive carcinoma (Figs. 2.26 and 2.27).

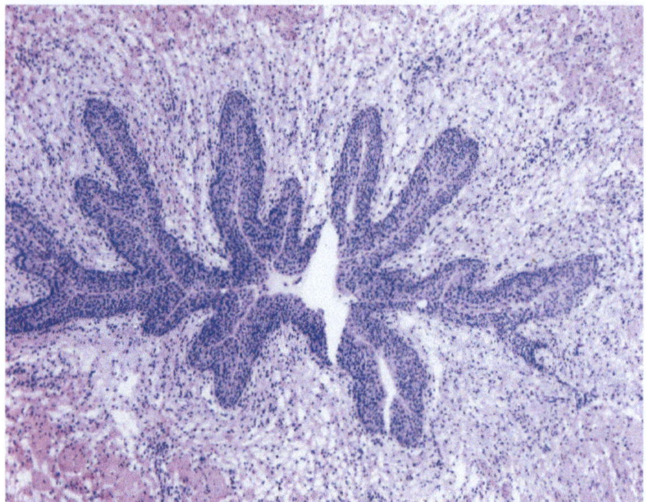

FIGURE 2.5 *Low-grade dysplasia of ureteral urothelium*. At low magnification, the urothelium appears slightly thickened with mild loss of cellular polarity. The diagnosis should be made with great caution. The subepithelial tissue shows mild to moderate chronic inflammation.

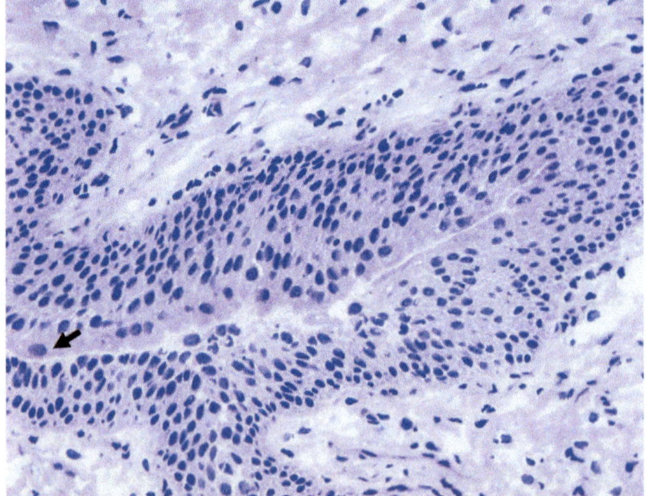

FIGURE 2.6 *Low-grade dysplasia of ureteral urothelium*. There is slight increase of urothelial cell layers and mild loss of polarity. The cells are mildly enlarged and appear hyperchromatic. There is also appreciable nuclear pleomorphism. The umbrella cell layer may still be intact (*arrow*).

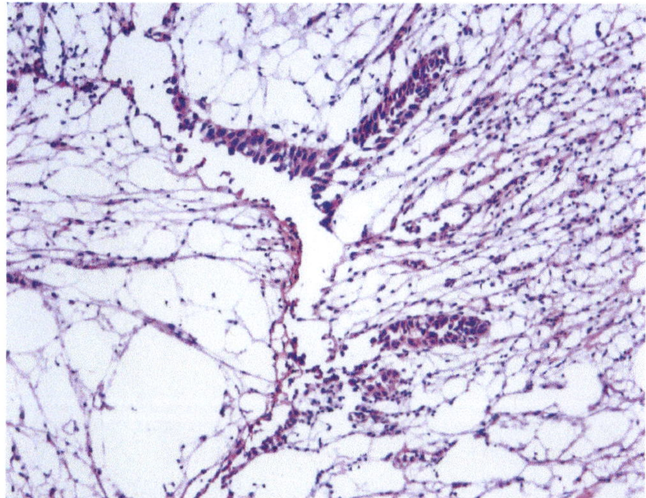

FIGURE 2.7 *High-grade dysplasia/carcinoma in situ*. The urothelium is partially denuded with marked edema of the subepithelial tissue. At low power, the remaining urothelium appears hyperchromatic.

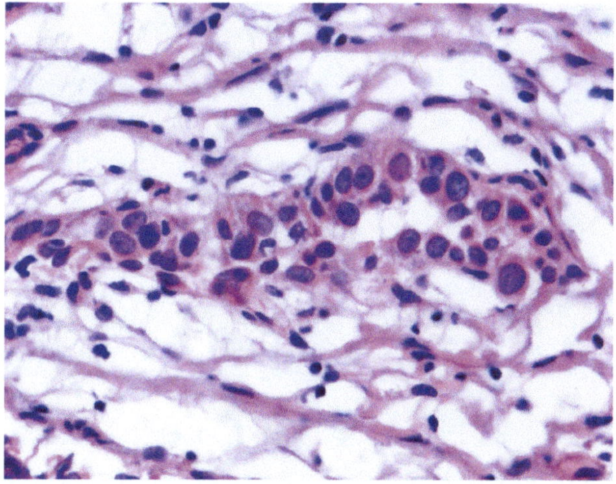

FIGURE 2.8 *High-grade dysplasia/carcinoma in situ*. Although there are only one or two layers of urothelial cells, these cells show marked nuclear enlargement, rounded nuclear contour, pleomorphism, and high N/C ratio, which are sufficient for a diagnosis of high-grade dysplasia or carcinoma in situ.

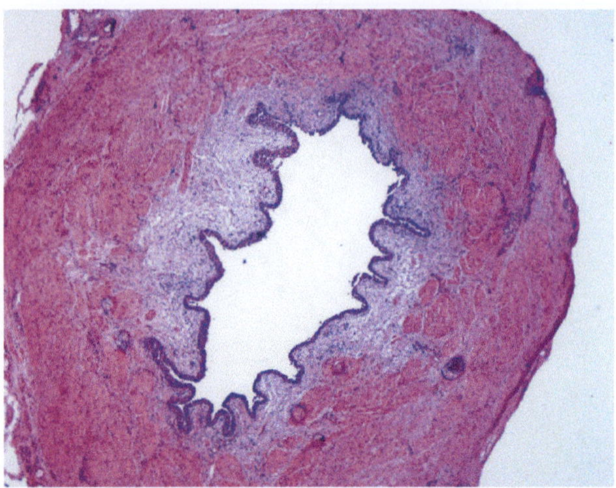

FIGURE 2.9 Low-power view showing a dilated ureter with thin urothelium and mild chronic inflammation within the subepithelial connective tissue, extending to the muscularis. High-grade dysplasia/carcinoma in situ is often associated with prominent chronic inflammation or fibrosis.

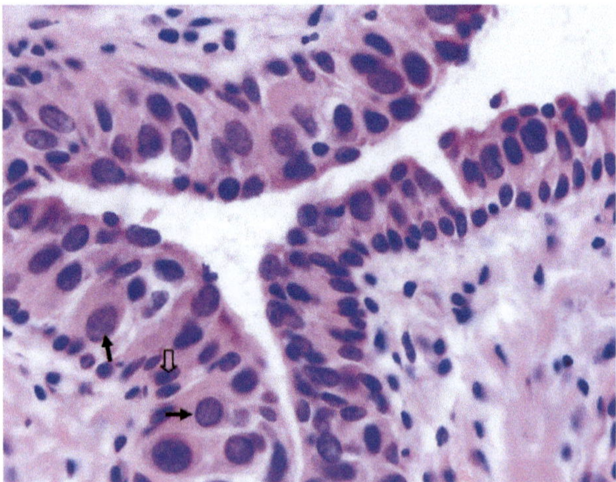

FIGURE 2.10 *High-grade dysplasia/carcinoma in situ.* High-power view showing urothelial cells with marked nuclear enlargement and pleomorphism. The tumor cells show pagetoid spread along the basement membrane and in between normal urothelial cells (*solid arrows*). Recognition of marked single cells or small groups of cells with high nuclear atypia by comparing with adjacent relatively normal urothelial cells (*open arrow*) is very helpful for the diagnosis.

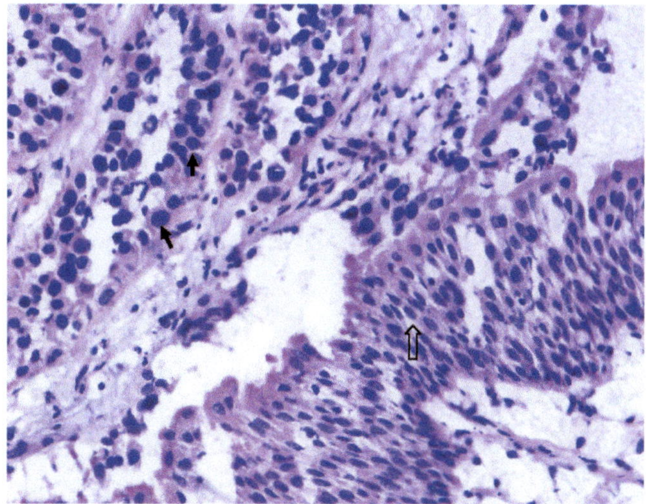

FIGURE 2.11 *High-grade dysplasia/carcinoma in situ*. Comparing to the relatively normal urothelial cells (*lower right, open arrow*), the lining epithelial cells and nests (*solid arrows*) on upper left corner show nuclear crowding, loss of polarity, rounded nuclei, marked hyperchromatia, increased N/C ratio, and increased mitoses and apoptosis.

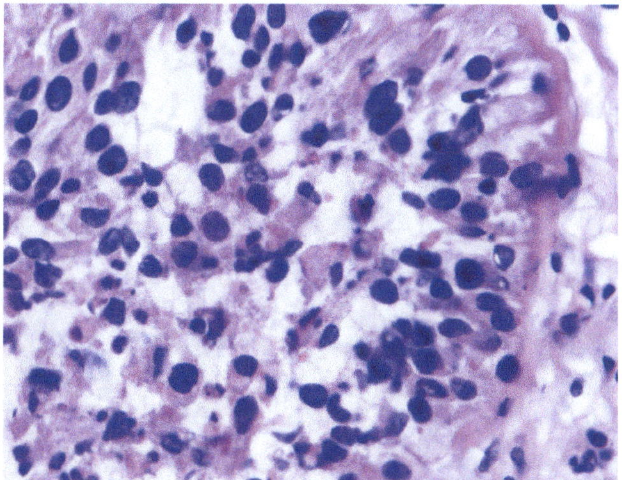

FIGURE 2.12 *High-grade dysplasia/carcinoma in situ*. High-power view showing nuclear crowding, loss of polarity, cells with rounded nuclei, pleomorphism, marked hyperchromatia, and single-cell necrosis.

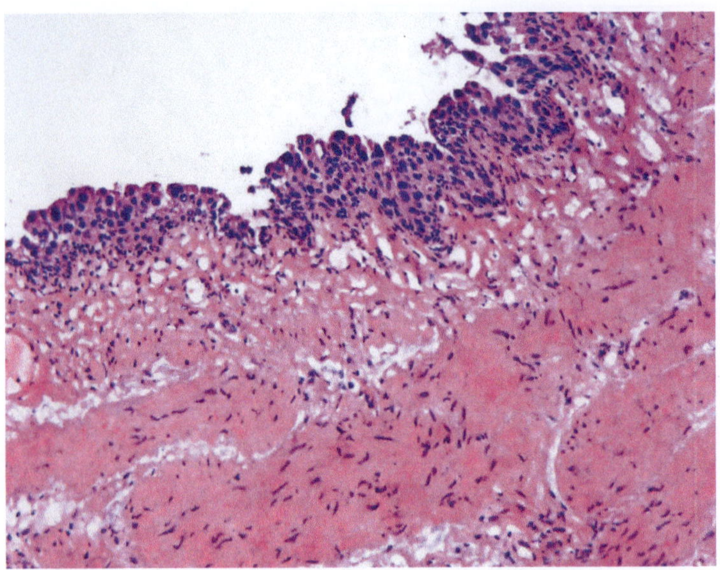

FIGURE 2.13 *High-grade dysplasia/carcinoma in situ.* Low-power view showing nuclear crowding, loss of polarity, and marked hyperchromatia.

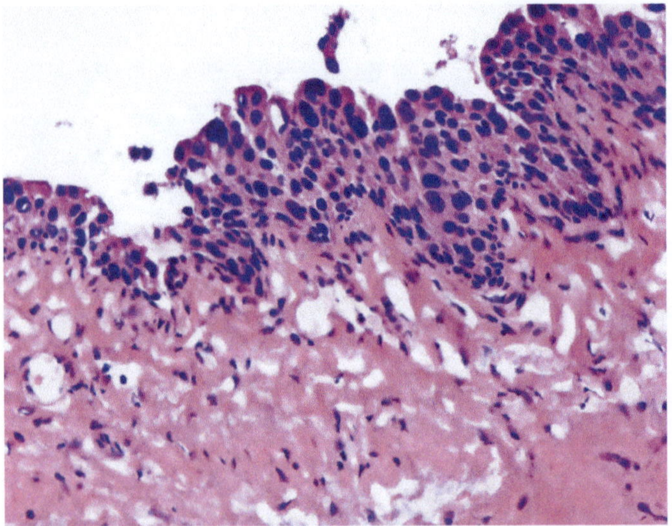

FIGURE 2.14 *High-grade dysplasia/carcinoma in situ.* High-power view showing full thickness severe dysplastic changes with nuclear crowding, loss of polarity, rounded nuclei, pleomorphism, and marked hyperchromatia.

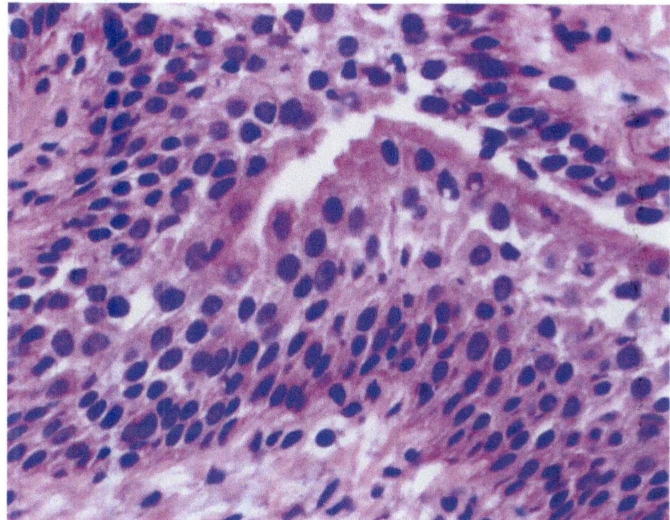

FIGURE 2.15 *Reactive atypia of ureteral urothelium.* There is preservation of cellular polarity and an intact layer of umbrella cells. The cells are relatively uniform and have smooth nuclear contour and small nucleoli.

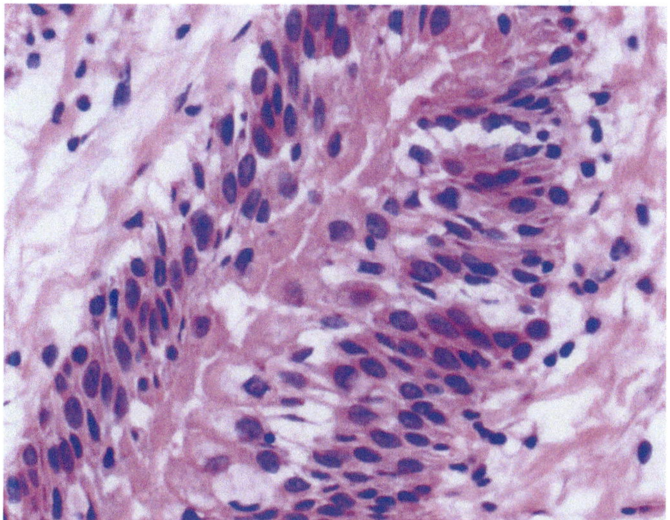

FIGURE 2.16 *Reactive atypia of ureteral urothelium.* High-power view showing preservation of cellular polarity and an intact layer of umbrella cells. The cells are uniformly enlarged and have small nucleoli.

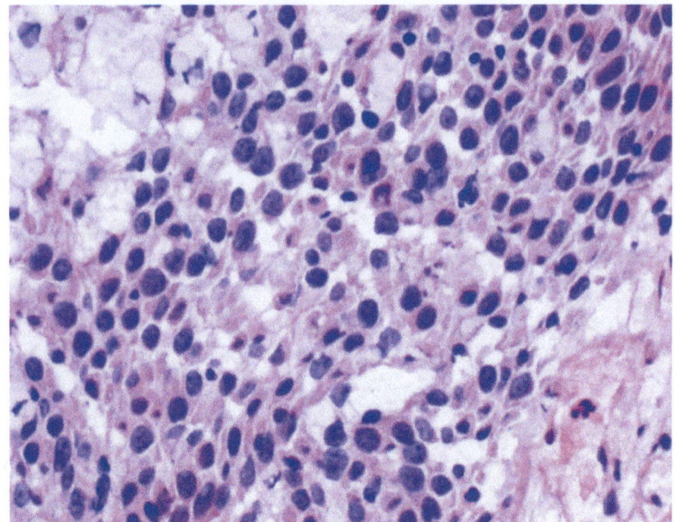

FIGURE 2.17 *Reactive atypia of ureteral urothelium.* Be aware of artifact causing compression of the ureteral lumen. All urothelial cells are relatively uniform with preserved polarity and small nucleoli.

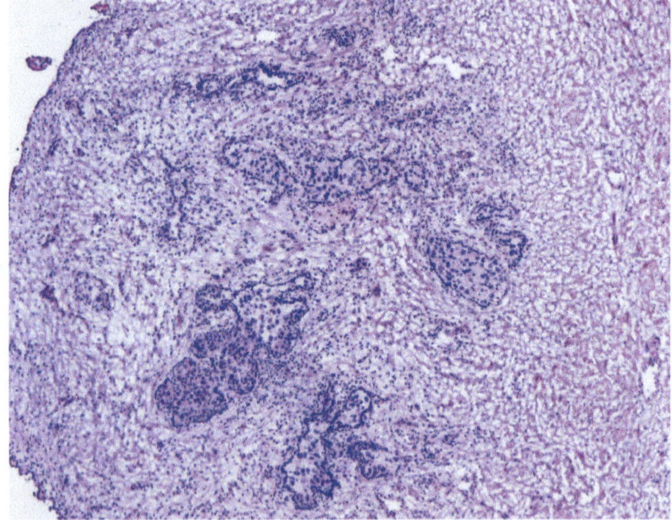

FIGURE 2.18 *Positive urethral margin with urothelial carcinoma in situ.* The periurethral ducts and glands are filled with highly atypical cells surrounded by chronic inflammation. The overlying surface urothelium (*left*) is frequently denuded.

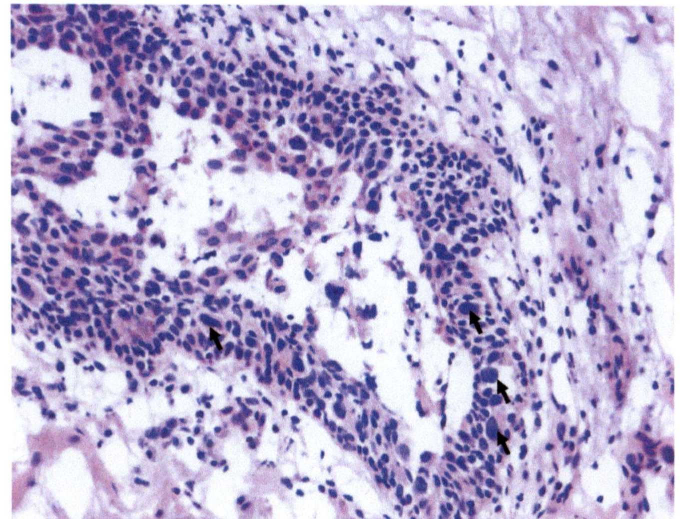

FIGURE 2.19 *Positive urethral margin with urothelial carcinoma in situ.* Large atypical cells with pagetoid spread within the urothelium of periurethral ducts (*arrows*).

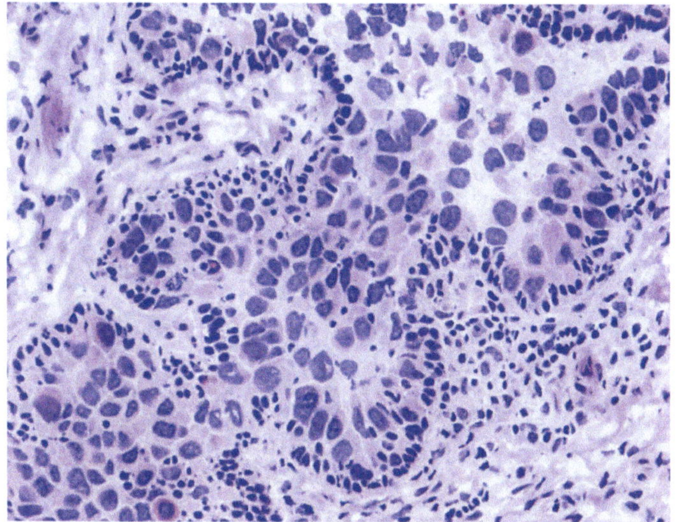

FIGURE 2.20 *Positive urethral margin with urothelial carcinoma in situ.* The periurethral ducts is replaced by highly atypical tumor cells with markedly enlarged and pleomorphic nuclei, frequent mitoses, and apoptosis. A rim of residual basal urothelial cells is present. The duct is surrounded by chronic inflammatory cells.

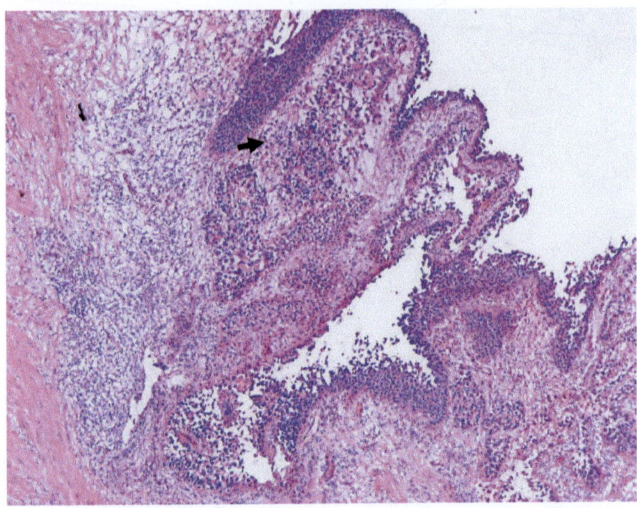

FIGURE 2.21 *Carcinoma in situ with superficial subepithelial invasion (arrow)*. Low-power viewing showing marked irregular contour of the urothelium with proliferation of nests of tumor cells within the subepithelial tissue and marked chronic inflammation.

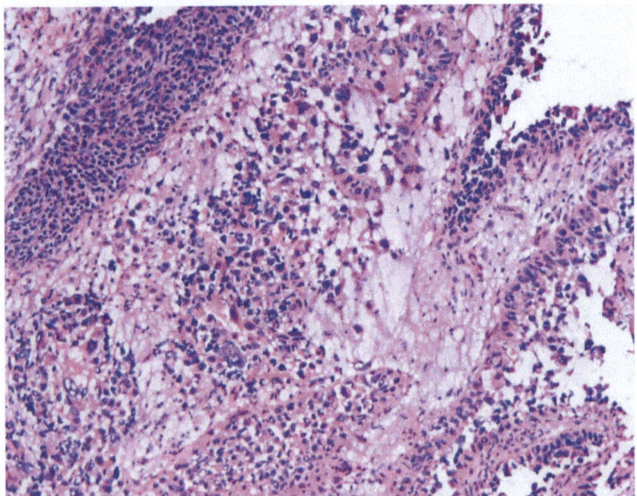

FIGURE 2.22 *Carcinoma in situ with superficial subepithelial invasion*. The nests of tumor cells show focal disruption of basement membrane and single cell invasion into the subepithelial connective tissue and desmoplastic/inflammatory reaction.

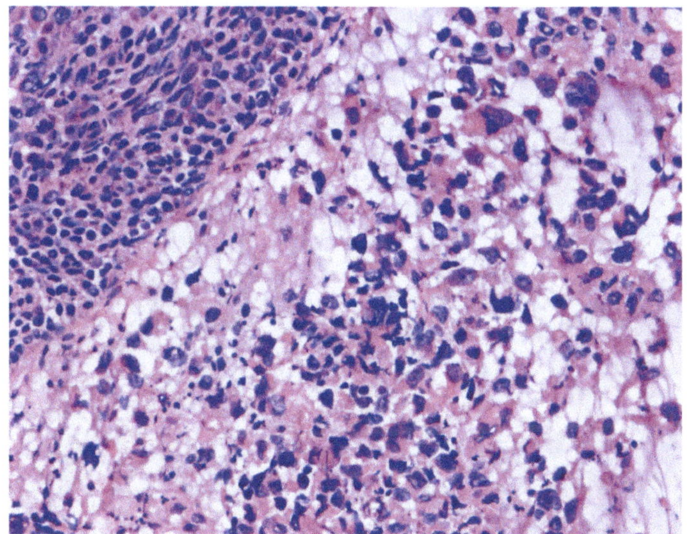

FIGURE 2.23 *Carcinoma in situ with superficial subepithelial invasion*. The nests of tumor cells show focal disruption of basement membrane and single cells invasion into the subepithelial connective tissue.

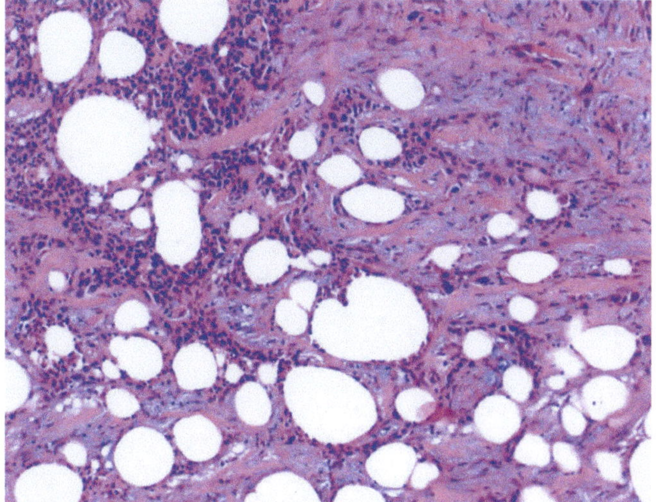

FIGURE 2.24 *Invasive urothelial carcinoma at the perivesical soft tissue margin*. Nests, cords, and single atypical cells infiltrating the fat with dense desmoplastic stroma.

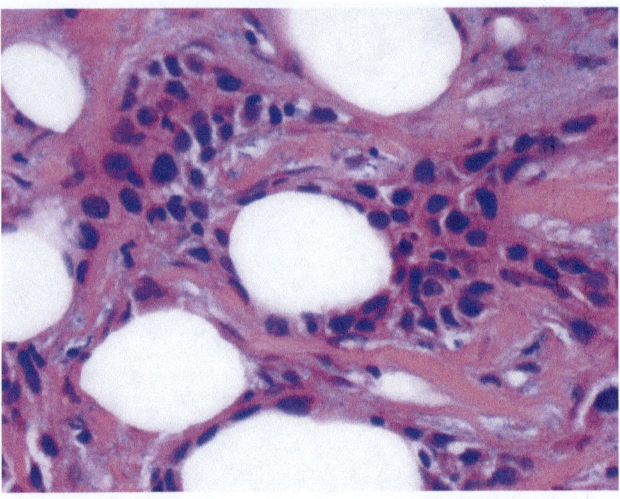

FIGURE 2.25 *Invasive urothelial carcinoma at the perivesical soft tissue margin*. Nests, cords, and single atypical cells with significant pleomorphism, hyperchromasia, and mitoses.

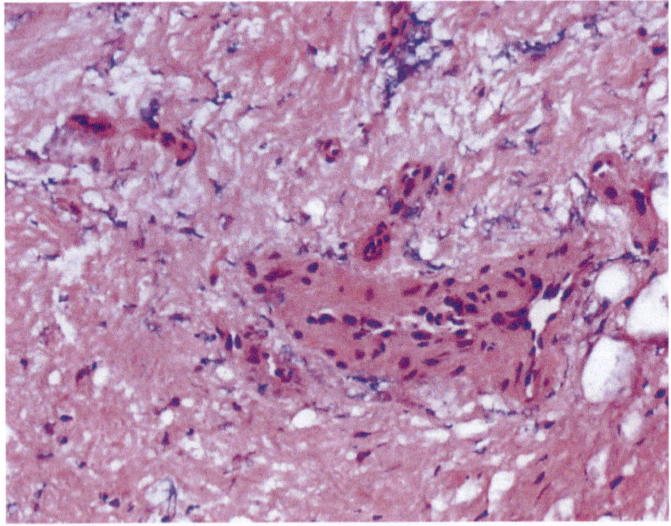

FIGURE 2.26 Reactive vessels with plump endothelial cells in frozen section simulating invasive carcinoma.

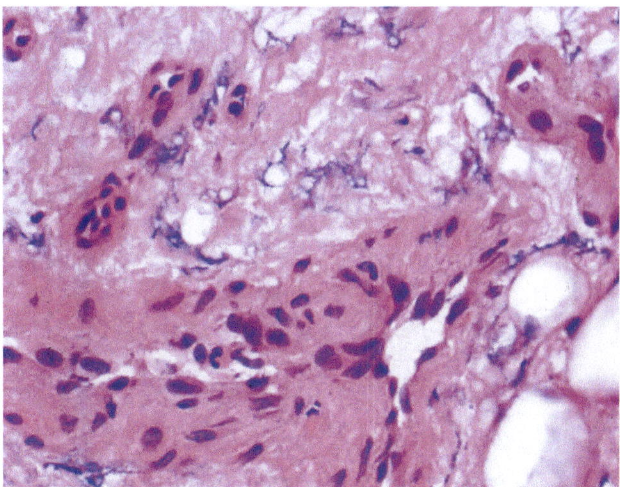

FIGURE 2.27 *Reactive blood vessels simulating carcinoma.* Note plump endothelial cells in frozen section. As compared with invasive carcinoma, these cells display low N/C ratio, homogeneous open chromatin, and no mitoses.

EVALUATION OF THE SURGICAL MARGINS DURING PARTIAL CYSTECTOMY

Clinical Background

The role of partial cystecomy is controversial and is reserved for highly selected patients. The most common indications for partial cystectomy include solitary tumor located in the dome of the bladder, tumor associated with bladder diverticulum, or urachal adenocarcinoma.[73] The challenges and selection criteria for patients for partial cystectomy are beyond the scope of this chapter.

Specimen Handling

The resection margin includes the entire mucosa and bladder wall of resection. Careful gross examination and communication with the surgeon are critical to identify the tumor and/or suspicious area. The choice of perpendicular or en face sections for FS evaluation depends on the distance of tumor and margin determined by careful gross examination and palpation. Ink should be applied to the entire resection margin before submission of FS. If tumor is near the resection margin, sections perpendicular to the resection margin can more accurately delineate the status of margin.

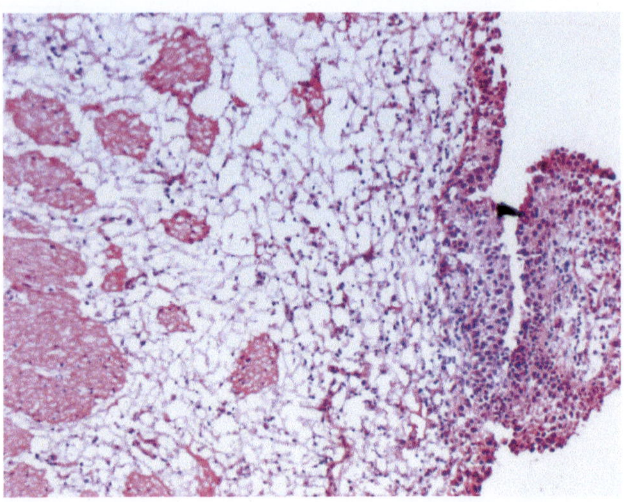

FIGURE 2.28. *En face margin of partial cystectomy specimen*: There are focal high-grade papillary carcinoma and carcinoma in situ at the margin.

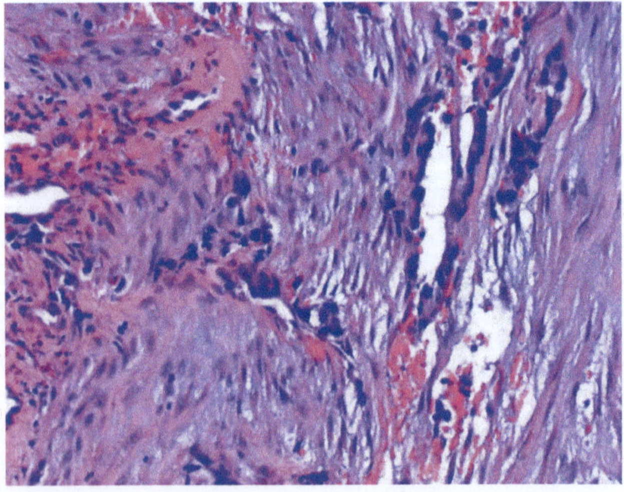

FIGURE 2.29 *Focal invasive carcinoma* is present at the subepithelial connective tissue resection margin of a partial cystectomy specimen. Nests and cords of tumor cells surrounded by marked desmoplasia.

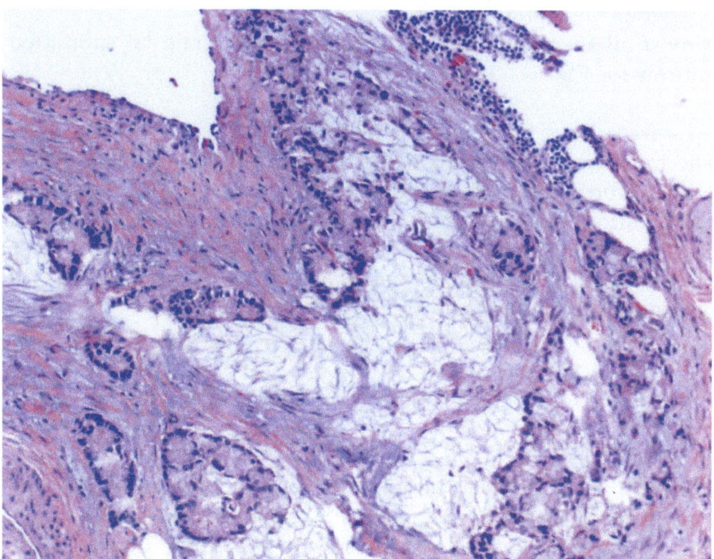

FIGURE 2.30 *Invasive urachal mucinous adenocarcinoma.* The tumor tissue is present at the perivesical resection margin of a partial cystectomy specimen. Intracytoplasmic mucin and pools of extracellular mucin are present.

Interpretation

The diagnosis of high-grade dysplasia/CIS and its pitfalls are similar to those for the ureteral and urethral margins. Invasive tumor in subepithelial tissue, muscularis propria, and perivesical fat can occasionally be seen (Figs. 2.28–2.30). Small focus of urachal adenocarcinoma of mucinous or signet ring cell type may show only intramural mucin pool; therefore, deep sections are often necessary to identify clusters of single tumor cells for a definitive diagnosis. If no tumor cells are identified on deep levels, this information should be clearly communicated with the surgeon.

EXTRAVESICAL OR BLADDER PERITONEAL NODULES OR MASSES

Clinical Background

During radical cystectomy, colorectal surgery, or gynecologic surgery, incidental lesions either in the form of peritoneal nodule, irregular thickening, or area of discoloration may be visualized on the bladder wall by surgeon. FS is often requested to identify the nature of these lesions. The diagnosis rarely changes the course of surgery, but may be part of the staging procedure.

Specimen Handling

Almost all specimens are small biopsy and should be submitted entirely for FS.

Interpretation

The most frequent diagnostic entities include mesothelial hyperplasia, fibrotic and hyalinized nodule, chronic inflammation, calcification, endometriosis, endocervicosis, endosalpingiosis, and, rarely, metastatic carcinoma. In these situations, awareness of the clinical history and histological features of these lesions will provide an accurate diagnosis.

FROZEN SECTION DIAGNOSIS OF BLADDER LESIONS

Clinical Background

Although most bladder tumors are biopsied preoperatively for a specific diagnosis and staging, FS diagnosis of bladder tumor may be rarely requested to provide an immediate diagnosis for selection of the surgical procedure. The reasons may also include unsuccessful previous biopsy or a need to secure adequate specimen for diagnosis and staging. This usually involves confirmatory diagnosis of bladder tumor and evaluating depth of invasion of a urothelial carcinoma. However, accurate typing of an unusual primary bladder tumor or differentiating urothelial carcinoma from prostatic or colonic adenocarcinoma extending to the bladder is also occasionally requested.

Specimen Handling

Small transurethral biopsy or resection specimens should be entirely submitted. If the specimen is composed of multiple fragments, selective pieces can be submitted. Muscularis propria tissue may be recognizable by careful gross examination and at least a portion of it should be submitted for FS. Communication with the surgeon with regard to the purpose of the FS request, impact of the diagnosis on the surgical approaches at hand, and possible limitation of FS is critical.

Interpretation

Over 90% of the bladder carcinomas in the USA are urothelial carcinomas, approximately 20% of which show divergent differentiation or variant morphology. Table 2.2 lists the WHO classification of invasive urothelial carcinoma and its variants, their incidences,

TABLE 2.2 WHO classification of invasive urothelial carcinoma and variants.

Infiltrating urothelial carcinoma and variants	Frequency (%)
Not otherwise specified	70–80
With squamous differentiation	10–20
With glandular differentiation	5–10
With trophoblastic differentiation	Rare
Nested	<1
Microcystic	<1
Micropapillary	1–5
Lymphoepithelioma-like	Rare
Plasmacytoid	Rare
Sarcomatoid	1–2
Giant cell	Rare
Undifferentiated	Rare

and main diagnostic features. Some common pitfalls for diagnosis and their differential diagnoses are listed in Table 2.3 (invasive carcinoma and differential diagnosis).

Squamous and glandular differentiation ranging from focal to extensive are the most common morphological variants of urothelial carcinoma and should not be misinterpreted as pure squamous cell carcinoma or adenocarcinoma because their prognosis and treatment might be different. In the case of urothelial carcinoma with glandular differentiation, the differential diagnoses should include *colonic adenocarcinoma invading the bladder, prostatic adenocarcinoma extending into the bladder,* or *a primary bladder adenocarcinoma,* in this order of incidence. Because primary adenocarcinomas of bladder and colon are often histologically similar, their distinction mainly depends on clinical information, imaging studies, and intraoperative examination. Prostatic adenocarcinoma may extend to the bladder neck and base. These tumors, usually of a high Gleason's score, may or may not display obvious glandular formation, but are composed of relatively uniform cells with round to oval nuclei, fine nuclear chromatin, prominent nucleoli, and relatively few mitoses. In contrast, nuclear pleomorphism with coarse chromatin and numerous mitoses are usual features of urothelial carcinoma. Comparison with the previous biopsy of the primary tumor, if available, is always helpful. Rare primary bladder adenocarcinomas are composed of signet ring cells and can be a diagnostic challenge at intraoperative FS, because this type of tumor may not form a

TABLE 2.3 Common bladder urothelial carcinoma variants, differential diagnoses, and their key diagnostic features.

	Differential diagnoses	Features favoring urothelial carcinoma variant
With squamous differentiation	Pure squamous cell carcinoma	Urothelial carcinoma NOS component; urothelial CIS
	Secondary or metastasis	Clinical history and surgical findings
With glandular differentiation	Primary adenocarcinoma	Urothelial carcinoma NOS component; urothelial CIS
	Urachal adenocarcinoma	Non-dome location; clinical findings
	Secondary or metastasis (colorectal or prostate)	Clinical history and surgical findings
Nested variant	von Brunn's nests	Urothelial carcinoma NOS component; urothelial CIS; deep invasion; more pronounced cytologic atypia
	Paraganglioma	NOS component; urothelial CIS
	Metastatic prostate carcinoma	More pronounced cytologic atypia and desmoplasia
	Nephrogenic adenoma	No inflammation; deeper location
Microcystic variant	Cystitis cystica/glandularis	Deeper location, greater cytologic atypia
	Nephrogenic adenoma	No inflammation; deeper location
	Primary or metastatic adenocarcinoma	Clinical history
Sarcomatoid carcinoma	Primary sarcoma	NOS carcinoma; CIS
	Postoperative spindle cell nodule	NOS carcinoma; CIS; greater cytologic atypia
	Inflammatory myofibroblastic tumor	NOS carcinoma; CIS; greater cytologic atypia
Micropapillary variant	Metastatic carcinoma	Clinical history
Small cell carcinoma	Lymphoma	Clinical history; NOS component; CIS
	Secondary or metastatic small cell carcinoma	Clinical history; urothelial carcinoma NOS, CIS
	Primary undifferentiated carcinoma	Smaller nuclei, less pleomorphic, positive neuroendocrine markers

mass, but tends to diffusely infiltrate the bladder wall as individual cells. Diagnosing nodal metastasis, which often occurs with this tumor type, may also be difficult on FS because the tumor cells may closely simulate sinusoidal histiocytes.

The depth of invasive urothelial carcinoma is best evaluated on permanent sections of preoperative transurethral biopsy or tumor resection specimen. Because invasion into muscularis propria is a major indication for radical cystectomy, the diagnosis must be accurate and differentiated from a tumor-induced desmoplastic myofibroblastic reaction or invasion into hyperplastic muscularis mucosae. It should be emphasized, however, that the differentiation may be impossible in small tissue samples, even in permanent sections. If called upon on evaluation of depth of tumor invasion on FS, unless it is obvious muscularis propria invasion, a conservative diagnosis should be made (Figs. 2.31–2.33). Muscularis propria invasion is recognized by tumor cells infiltrating large bundles of unequivocal smooth muscle fibers, which appear as closely packed arrangements of spindled cells with cigar-shaped nuclei and abundant eosinophilic cytoplasm (Figs. 2.34–2.36). It is differentiated from tumor-induced desmoplastic reaction, which

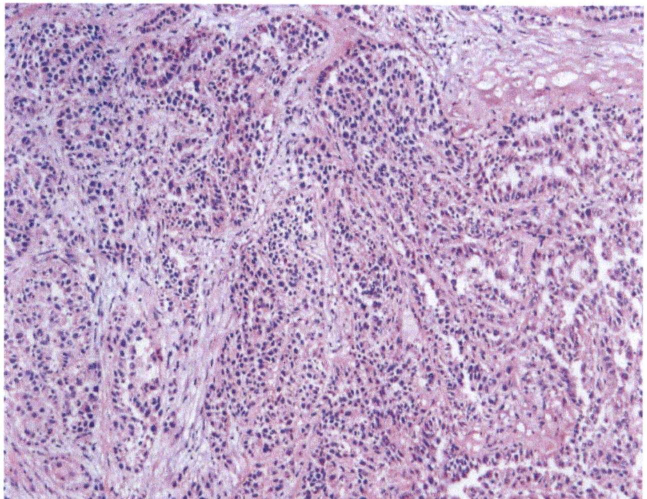

FIGURE 2.31 *Invasive urothelial carcinoma invading the subepithelial tissue.* Large sheets and nests of tumor cells infiltrating the stroma with desmoplastic reaction.

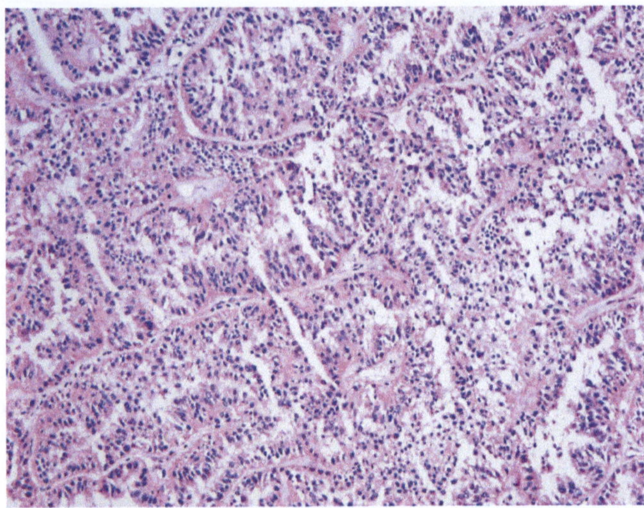

FIGURE 2.32 *Urothelial carcinoma with a confluent growth pattern with scanty stroma.* Although the findings may be suspicious for invasive carcinoma, evaluation of other areas is necessary to make the final diagnosis of invasion.

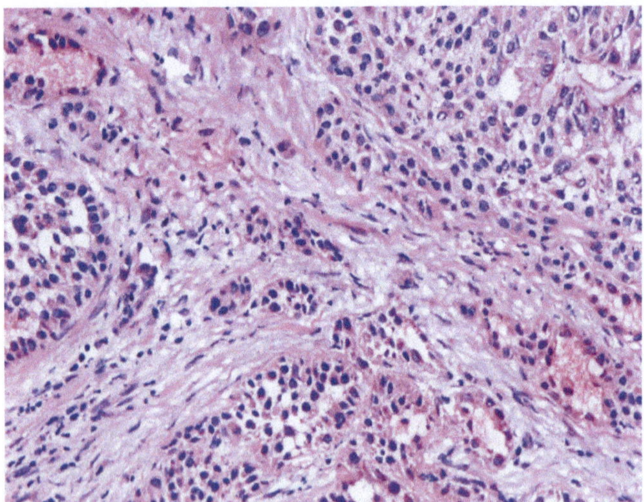

FIGURE 2.33 *Invasive urothelial carcinoma* invades into stromal tissue with small clusters and a few single tumor cells with desmoplastic reaction.

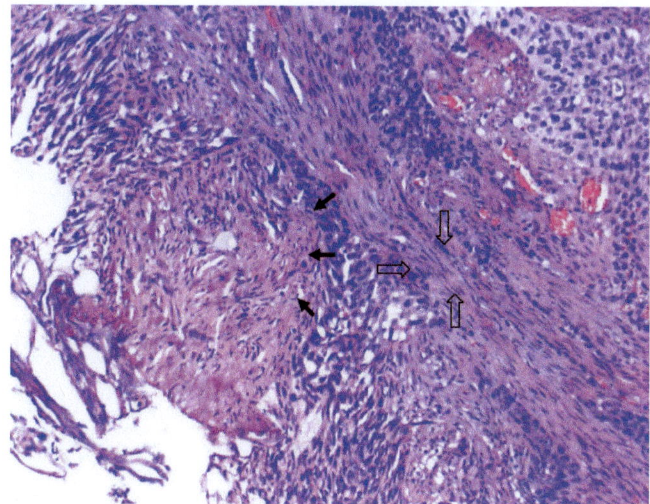

FIGURE 2.34 *Invasive urothelial carcinoma* with sheets of cauterized tumor cells surrounding bundles of smooth muscle cells of muscularis propria (*solid arrows*). Desmoplasia is also present. (*open arrows*).

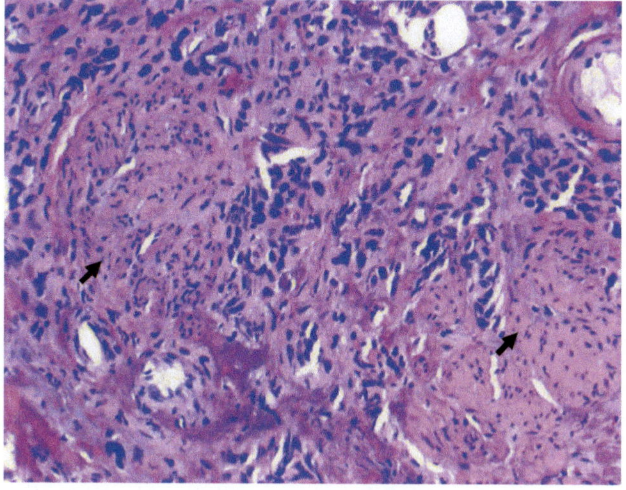

FIGURE 2.35 *Invasive urothelial carcinoma* with irregular nests of tumor cells infiltrating into large bundles of muscularis propria (*arrows*). On frozen section, these changes may be seen focally.

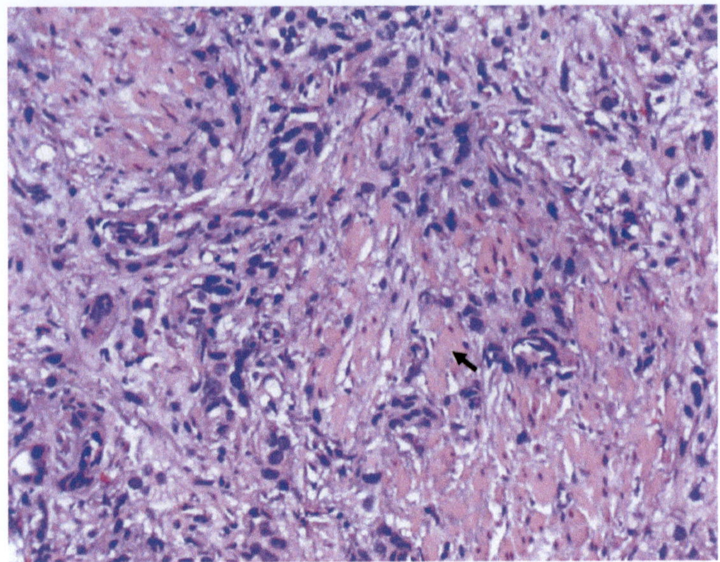

FIGURE 2.36 *Invasive urothelial carcinoma* with irregular nests of tumor cells, dissecting and destroying bundles of smooth muscles of muscularis propria (*arrow*). The smooth muscle cells have small spindle nuclei and abundant dense eosinophilic cytoplasm, which is different from that of myofibroblasts.

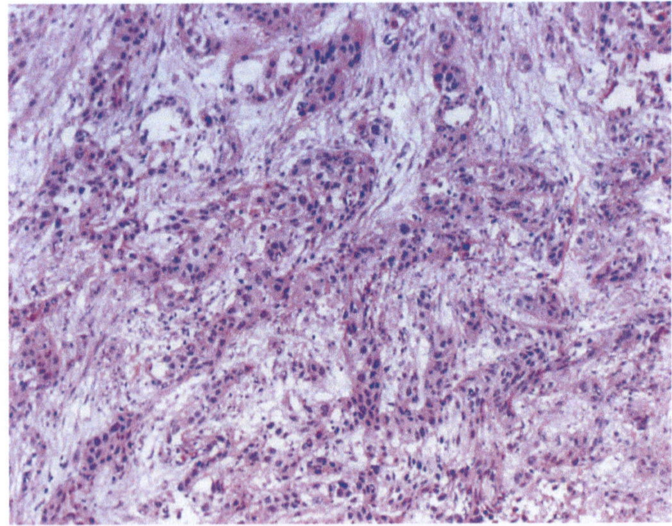

FIGURE 2.37 *Invasive urothelial carcinoma* with irregular nests of tumor cells infiltrating subepithelial tissue with fibroblastic reaction, edema, and chronic inflammation. The myofibroblasts usually have elongated spindle and pointed nuclei and cytoplasmic processes.

may include abundant myofibroblasts, by noting that the myofibroblasts usually have pointed nuclei, less eosinophilic cytoplasm than smooth muscle cells, and are usually separated by fibrous stroma (Fig. 2.37). Invasion to muscularis mucosae is usually suggested by the association of tumor cells with unequivocal but small and discontinuous smooth muscle bundles, which are close to large blood vessels.

Occasionally, an intraoperative diagnosis of fibroepithelial polyp or papilloma may abort the need of more radical procedure.

FROZEN SECTION DIAGNOSIS OF BLADDER NECK TISSUE IN RADICAL PROSTATECTOMY FOR PROSTATE ADENOCARCINOMA

Clinical Background

Bladder neck tissue is occasionally submitted for FS to check for the involvement by prostatic adenocarcinoma during radical prostatectomy. If positive, additional tissue might be obtained to achieve a negative margin if clinically feasible. Currently, involvement of bladder neck by prostate adenocarcinoma is considered to be high stage T4 tumor, although many recent studies dispute this conclusion.

Specimen Handling

The specimen is usually small and should be submitted entirely for FS.

Interpretation

The diagnosis is usually not a problem, as the tumor is more often high-grade tumor with large sheets of cribriform glands or fused glands, and diagnostic features of prostate carcinoma including large nuclei, prominent nucleoli, and lack of basal cells (Fig. 2.38). High-grade prostatic adenocarcinoma, particularly the ductal endometrioid adenocarcinoma, can present as bladder tumor in the bladder neck clinically, grossly and microscopically. Occasionally prostatic hyperplasia can present as bladder neck nodules. Microscopically, it displays nodular proliferation of mixed gland and stromal elements with no cytologic features of carcinoma. Occasionally small glandular hyperplasia (atypical adenomatous hyperplasia or adenosis) or pure hyperplastic stromal nodule can be seen as well.

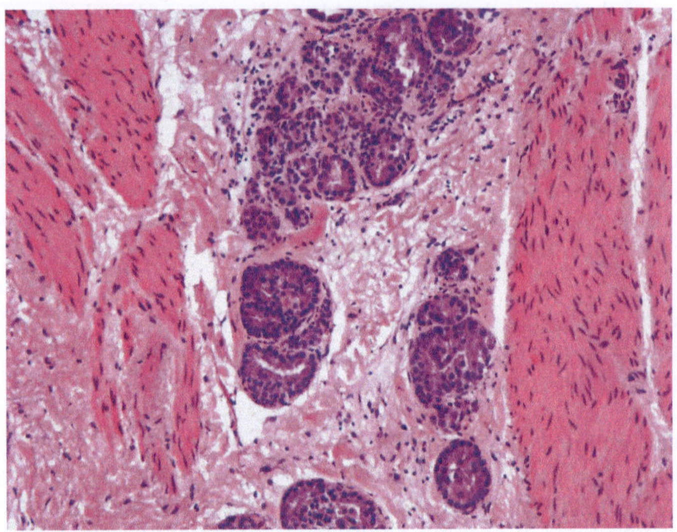

FIGURE 2.38 *Prostatic adenocarcinoma*. Gleason score 3 + 4 infiltrating through the bladder neck muscle bundles.

EVALUATION OF THE LYMPH NODES DURING CYSTECTOMY

Clinical Background

Bilateral pelvic lymph node dissection is a part of standard procedure of radical cystectomy for muscle invasive bladder carcinoma. Recently some investigators recommend extending the node dissection to the aortic bifurcation or the inferior mestenteric artery to include the common iliac and pre-sacral lymph nodes. FS examination is highly accurate in detecting nodal metastasis in patients with bladder cancer undergoing radical cystectomy and pelvic nodal dissection.[74,75] Evaluation of metastatic status of lymph nodes may have an immediate role in the intraoperative management decision making in terms of extent of nodal dissection or rarely termination of radical procedure.

Specimen Handling

Pelvic nodal dissection specimens are submitted either in block or in packets. Identification of lymph nodes is achieved by visual examination, palpation, and removal of fat tissue by blunt dissection. Representative sections from grossly metastatic lymph nodes are submitted, but lymph nodes that are grossly negative should be cut into thin slices of 2–3 mm and submitted entirely for microscopic examination if requested. The decision of performing intraoperative FS diagnosis of nodal metastasis should be made by close communication between the surgeons and the pathologists in advance or intraoperatively.

Interpretation

In conventional urothelial carcinoma, metastatic foci are usually not difficult to identify. However, small focus of poorly differentiated carcinoma or unusual tumor variants such as micropapillary, plamacytoid, or lymphoma-like carcinoma can be extremely subtle and easy to miss on FS (Figs. 2.39–2.42). Review of presurgical biopsy material and awareness of the variant histological types will be helpful. Careful examination of all submitted tissue and particular attention to the subcapsular sinus are important to avoid false negative diagnosis. On the contrary, histiocytic reaction characterized by sheet of histiocytes with abundant, granular cytoplasm replacing large portions of the pelvic lymph nodes is frequently seen in patients with joint prosthesis of the lower extremities, and should be differentiated from metastatic carcinoma (*see also* Chap. 4).

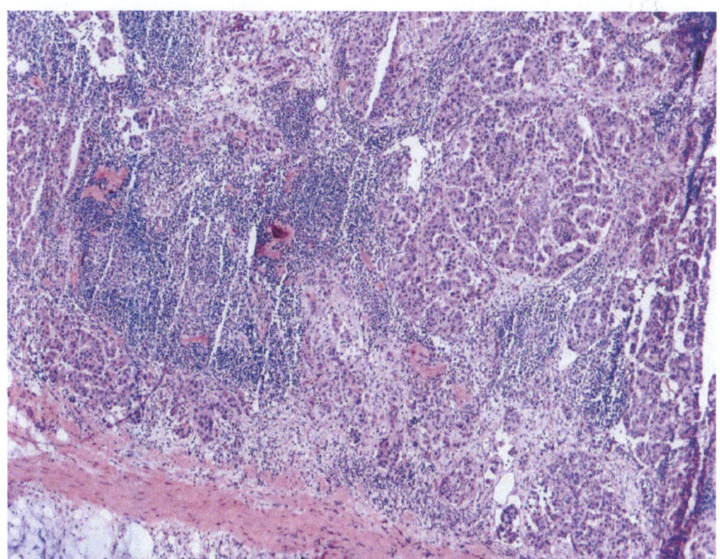

FIGURE 2.39 *Pelvic lymph node with metastatic urothelial carcinoma.* Large and small nests of carcinoma cells present in the subcapsular and medullary sinuses.

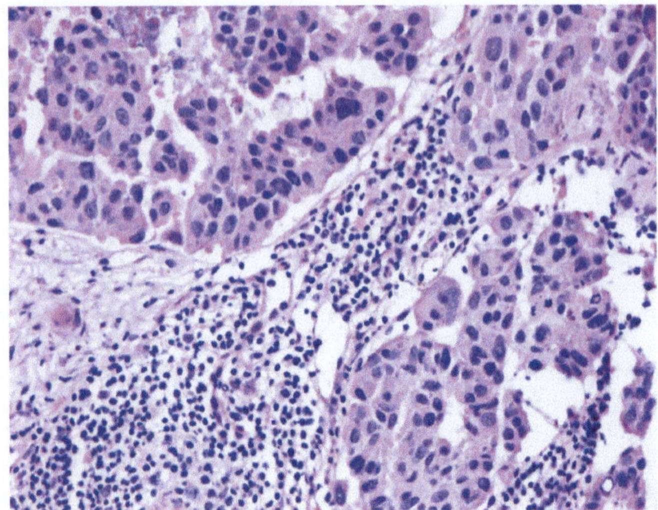

FIGURE 2.40 *Pelvic lymph node with metastatic urothelial carcinoma.* Nests of urothelial carcinoma within the nodal sinuses.

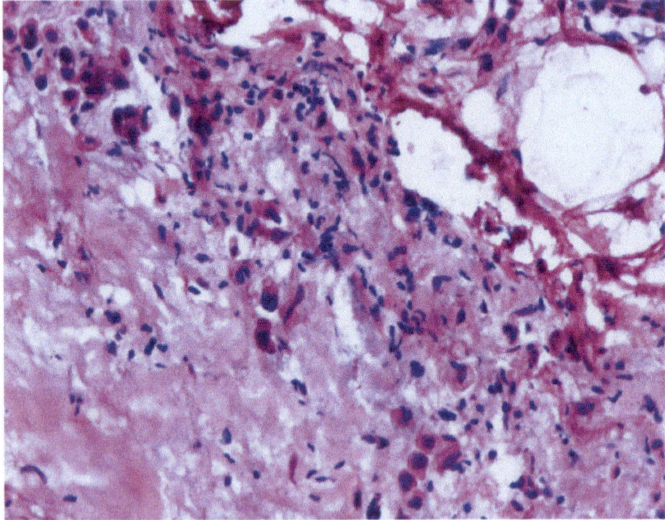

FIGURE 2.41 *Pelvic lymph node with metastatic urothelial carcinoma.* The lymph node is replaced by fibrosis and a few small clusters of atypical cells. This patient received neoadjuvant therapy before cystectomy and pelvic nodal dissection.

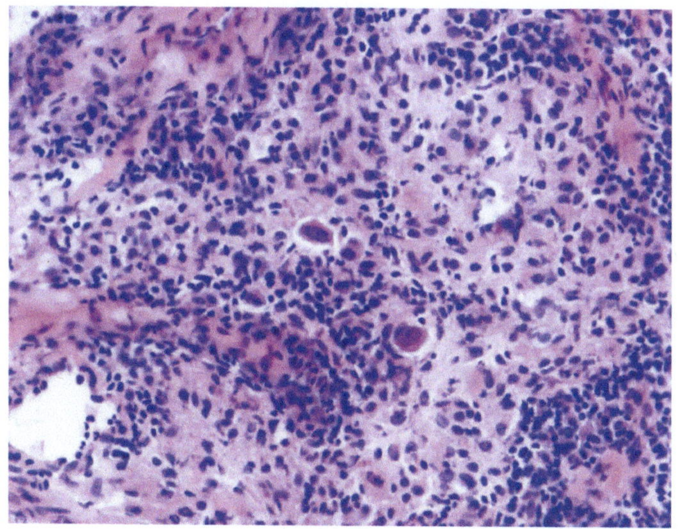

FIGURE 2.42 *Pelvic lymph node with metastatic urothelial carcinoma.* Two highly atypical tumor cells are present within the lymph node.

Chapter 3
Penis

Steven S. Shen, Luan D. Truong, and Jae Y. Ro

INDICATIONS FOR INTRAOPERATIVE PATHOLOGY CONSULTATION

The two main indications for intraoperative FS for penile cancer are margin evaluation for partial or total penectomies and nodal status evaluation. It has been shown that the use of intraoperative FS can lead to a concomitant decrease in both positive surgical margins and recurrence in squamous cell carcinoma or Paget's disease.[76, 77] Nowadays, the diagnosis of penile cancer is made almost exclusively by tissue biopsy before definitive surgery. In fact, using FS for the purpose of diagnosis at the time of surgery is discouraged because it is often difficult or impossible to make a distinction between a well-differentiated squamous cell carcinoma or verucous carcinoma from nonneoplastic conditions.

EVALUATION OF THE SURGICAL MARGINS FOR PARTIAL OR TOTAL PENECTOMY SPECIMENS

Clinical Background

Partial or total penectomy is an effective treatment for invasive squamous cell carcinoma of the penis. The goal is to ensure oncological control with negative resection margin. Tumor location, size, and depth of invasion help to determine the surgical management of the primary lesion. Intraoperative FS of proximal resection margin is often requested to ensure adequacy of resection. The margins that need to be evaluated during partial or total penectomy include: (1) skin margin, (2) corpora cavernosa and corpus spongiosum soft tissue margin, and (3) urethral margin. It is generally recommended that tumor excision with a 1.5–2.5 cm macroscopic surgical

L.D. Truong et al., *Frozen Section Library: Genitourinary Tract,*
Frozen Section Library 2, DOI 10.1007/978-1-4419-0691-5_3,
© Springer Science + Business Media, LLC 2009

TABLE 3.1 Primary site and frequency of penile squamous cell carcinoma (adapted from Ro JY et al. Urologic Surgical Pathology, 2nd Edition).

Site(s)	Frequency (%)
Glans	48
Prepuce	21
Coronal sulcus	6
Shaft	2
Glans and prepuce	9
Glans, prepuce, and shaft	14

margin is an attempt to minimize the local recurrence. Most of the squamous cell carcinomas arise from glans, prepuce, or coronal sulcus (Table 3.1). The carcinoma in situ can spread to the urethral mucosa, or rarely penile skin. The invasive carcinoma often directly invades into corpus spongiosum and corpora cavernosa. In addition to direct invasion, poorly differentiated squamous cell carcinoma or basaloid carcinoma can have lymphovascular invasion as well. For well-differentiated squamous cell carcinoma, verrucous carcinoma, or papillary squamous cell carcinoma, the chance of having a positive margin is very low. Urothelial carcinoma of penile urethra is exceedingly rare. Margin evaluation for this type of carcinoma includes carcinoma in situ of urethra, periurethral glands involvement, or invasion carcinoma involving corpus spongiosum and corpora cavernosa. The most common diagnostic pitfalls and difficulties are discussed below.

Specimen Handling

Specimen is oriented and tumor is visually localized or palpated. The penile carcinomas are either exophytic/fungating or ulcerated/infiltrative. On the basis of the gross impression of cancer in relation to the margin, the manner of section submitted for FS will differ. For majority of the partial or total penectomy specimen, en face shaved margins are taken for FS. These margins include urethra, corpora cavernosa and corpus spongiosum with adjacent soft tissue, and skin tissue. When tumor is located near the margin by gross evaluation, the resection margin should be inked, and perpendicular sections of tumor with inked margin are better to evaluate its status and distance to that margin. Occasionally, small separate margin tissue is submitted by surgeon and this tissue should be entirely submitted for FS. If orientation with indicated margin (ink or suture) is provided, ink should be applied to the true margin; perpendicular sections with the inked margin should be taken and entirely submitted.

Interpretation

In most cases, the margin evaluation is not difficult for the well-differentiated carcinoma (warty or verrucous) because their growth pattern is distinct from normal tissue. The margin of resection is rarely positive. Normal penile skin has squamous lining with or without hyperkeratosis and delicate fibroconnective lamina propria (Fig. 3.1). Familiarity with penile urethral lining, squamous metaplasia, periurethral mucinous glands, as well as cavernosa tissue is helpful for correct interpretation of proximal tissue margins (Figs. 3.2–3.5). For poorly differentiated squamous carcinoma or basaloid carcinoma, deep stromal invasion or lymphovascular invasion is more likely to occur; therefore, in addition to skin and mucosa and urethra margin, careful examination of corpus spongiosum, corpora cavernosa, as well as lamina propia is necessary (Figs. 3.6 and 3.7). In general, almost all the penile lesions are diagnosed by preoperative

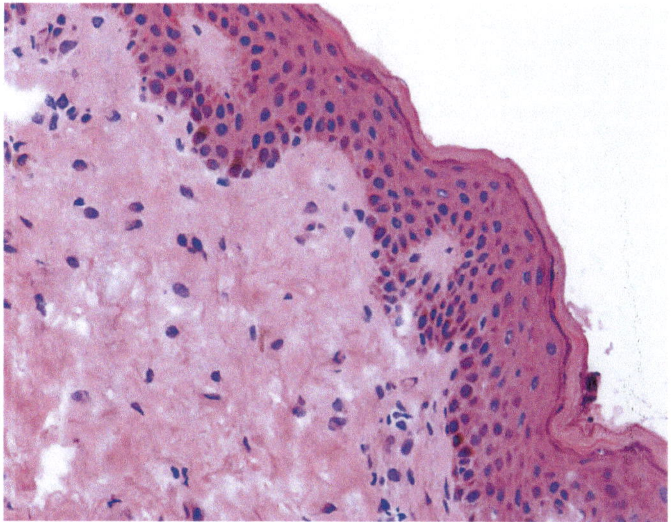

FIGURE 3.1 *Normal penile (glans) squamous mucosa with lamina propria fibroconnective tissue.* Mild hyperkeratosis is noted. There is abundant melanin pigmentation of the basal layers. No significant inflammation is present.

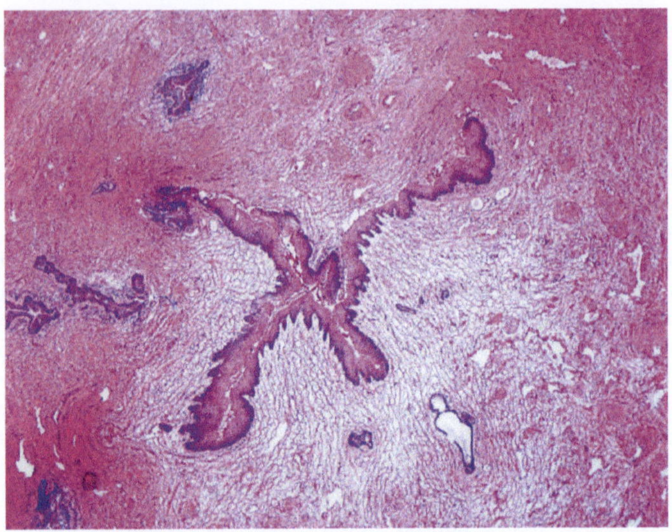

FIGURE 3.2 *Penile urethral margin.* A cross section of proximal urethral margin shows squamous lining, periurethral ducts within loose, edematous subepithelial tissue.

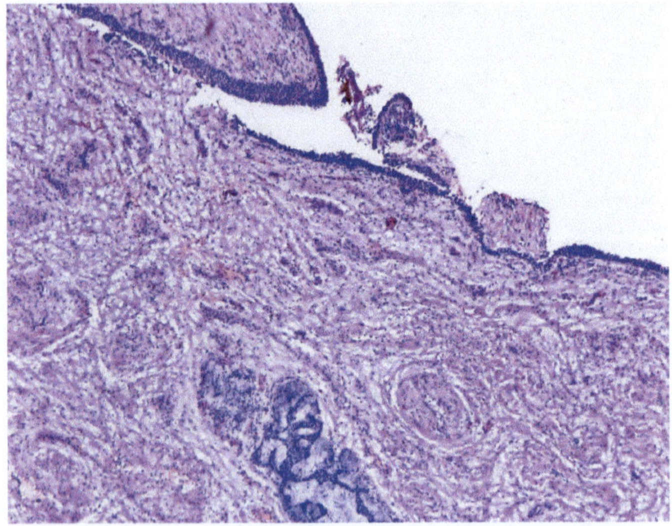

FIGURE 3.3 *Proximal normal urethral margin with urothelial lining and fibromuscular connective tissue.* A focus of mucinous glands and ducts is present in the lamina propria.

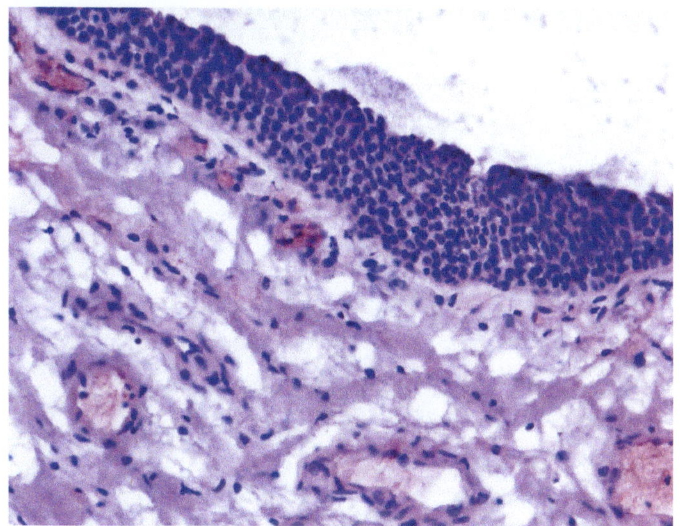

FIGURE 3.4 *Normal Penile urethra*. Penile urethra is lined by layers of urothelial cells with relatively monotonous cells, which are evenly distributed with preservation of polarity. No significant cytologic atypia, hyperplasia, or mitoses are present. The lamina propria tissue is composed of delicate fibrovascular tissue. On frozen section, a thicker section may show higher cellularity, and prolonged staining may affect the chromatin characteristic as well. These may lead to misinterpreting normal penile urethra as dysplastic change.

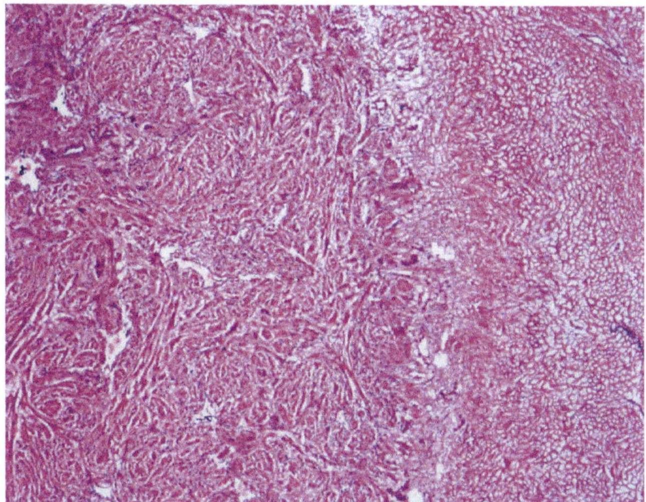

FIGURE 3.5 *Cross section of proximal resection margin of corpus carvernosum and tunica albuginea (right)*. The corpus carvernosum is composed of bundles of smooth muscle cells and abundant ectatic venous vessels.

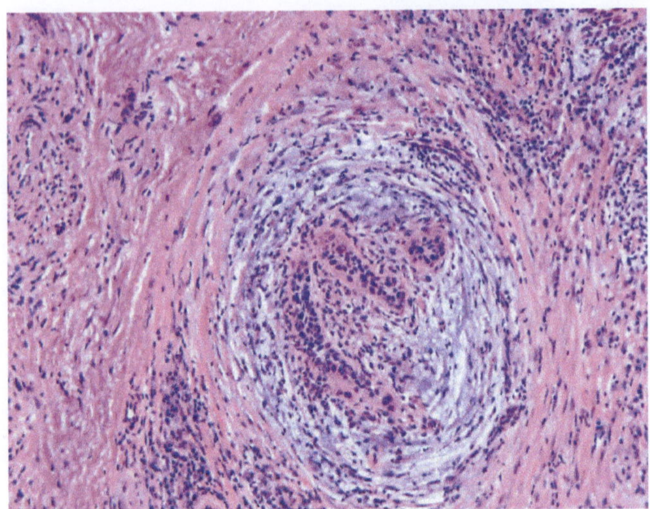

FIGURE 3.6 *Positive penile resection margin.* A focus of invasive squamous cell carcinoma at the proximal penile resection margin of lamina propria. Nests of tumor cells surrounded by desmoplastic and inflammatory reaction.

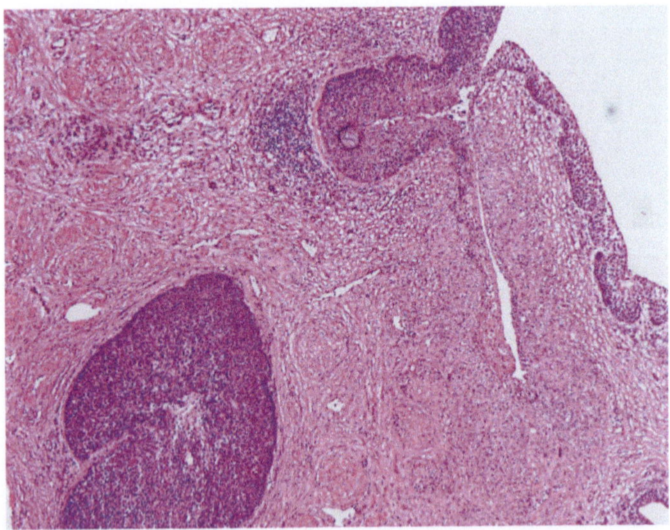

FIGURE 3.7 *Positive penile resection margin.* A large nest of basaloid squamous cell carcinoma within the distal portion of corpus spongiosum.

biopsy, and intraoperative diagnosis is usually not requested. Confirmatory FS diagnosis and tumor grading as well as evaluation of depth of invasion are requested for guidance of nodal dissection. A comparison of clinicopathological features of invasive squamous cell carcinoma and its variants is shown in Table 3.2. It should be noted that there are a number of situations in which a definitive diagnosis on FS is very difficult, even on permanent sections. Some of the most common difficult differentiation diagnoses on FS and their helpful features are discussed below.

Reactive hyperplasia versus squamous cell carcinoma in situ: In contrast to normal squamous epithelium, reactive hyperplasia can show prominent thickening of the epithelium, enlargement of nuclei, and occasional mitoses. Features that favor reactive hyperplasia include uniform nuclear enlargement and small nucleoli, spongiosis, intraepithelial and interface inflammatory cell infiltrate (Figs. 3.8 and 3.9). In contrast, carcinoma in situ shows full thickness dysplastic changes with increased N/C ratio, nuclear pleomorphism and mitoses, and lack of maturation (Figs. 3.10 and 3.11).

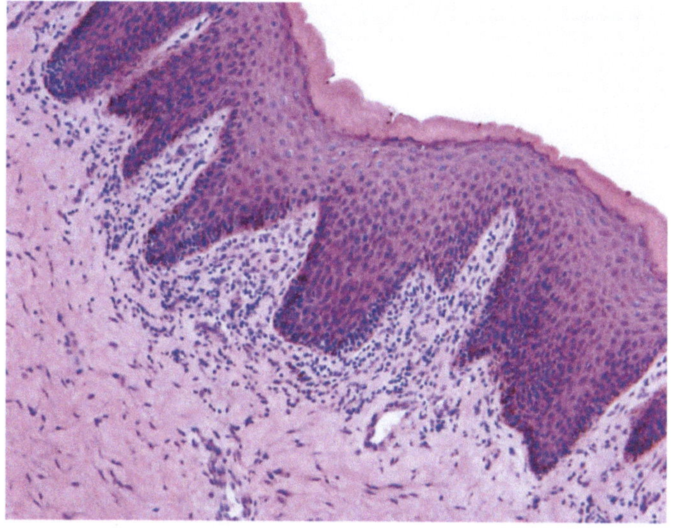

FIGURE 3.8 *Negative penile skin margin of a partial penectomy specimen.* There is mild hyperkeratosis, mild squamous hyperplasia, prominent subepithelial, and mild intraepithelial chronic inflammation. No significant cytologic atypia is present.

TABLE 3.2 Clinicopathological features of penile squamous cell carcinoma and variants.

	NOS	Basaloid	Warty	Verrucous	Sarcomatoid
Age (mean years)	60	55	61	50	60
Size (cm)	up to 14.0	>4.0	4.0	3.0	5.0–7.0
HPV-related	No	Yes	Yes	No	No
Koilocytosis	Absent	Absent	Prominent	Absent	Absent
Fibrovascular core	Present	Rare	Present	Rare	Absent
Pleomorphism	Marked	Moderate	Moderate	Mild	Marked
Mitoses	Frequent	Frequent	Occasional	Rare	Frequent
Keratinization	Variable	Absent	Present	Present	Absent
Base of lesion	Irregular jagged	Irregular infiltrative	Rounded or irregular	Regular, pushing	Irregular, jagged

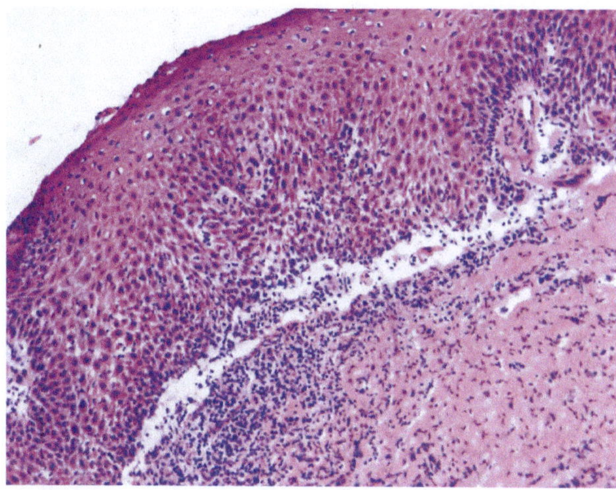

FIGURE 3.9 *Squamous hyperplasia and reactive atypia*. Penile skin resection margin showing marked squamous hyperplasia, spongiosis, and prominent dense chronic inflammation extending to the epithelium. Uniform nuclear enlargement and small nucleoli are characteristic.

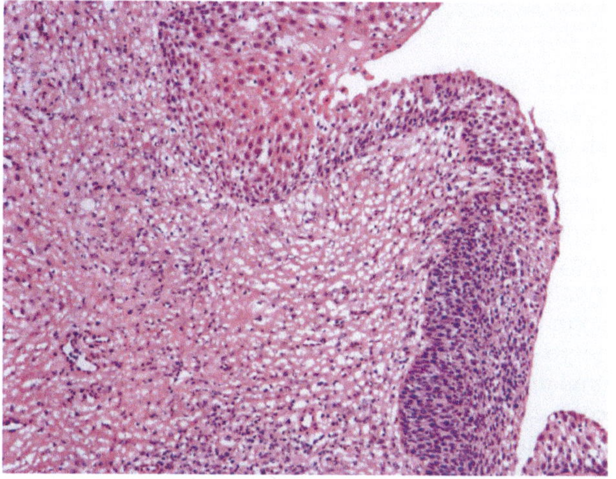

FIGURE 3.10 *Perpendicular section of margin with adjacent squamous cell carcinoma*. The nondysplastic squamous epithelium (*upper*) exhibits marked spongiosis, reactive atypia, and intraepithelial lymphocytes. The squamous cell carcinoma in situ (*lower*) is characterized by full thickness dysplasia with lack of maturation, high N/C ratio, and marked hyperchromatia of nuclei.

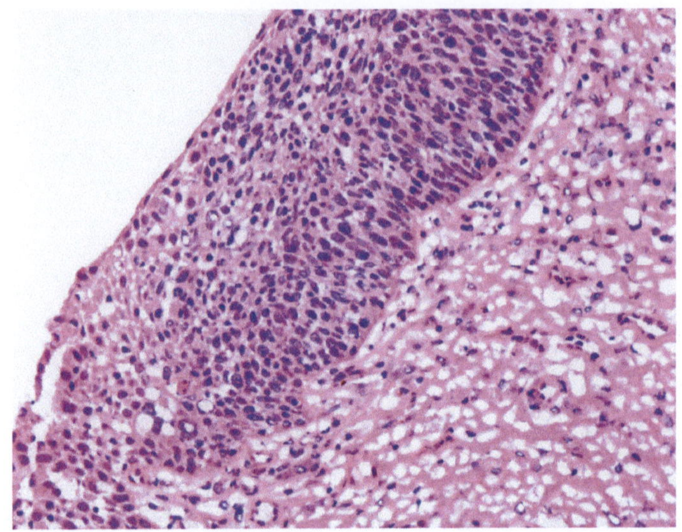

FIGURE 3.11 *Squamous cell carcinoma in situ.* There is marked increase of cellularity, lack of cytoplasmic maturation, increase of N/C ratio, nuclear enlargement, hyperchromasia, and significant pleomorphism.

Verrucous carcinoma versus well-differentiated squamous carcinoma versus hyperplasia: Verrucous carcinoma is characterized by high degree of cellular differentiation and lack of significant cytologic atypia and a pushing, blunt deep border with subepithelial stroma (Figs. 3.12–3.14). There can be chronic inflammation in the surrounding stroma but no desmoplastic reaction occurs. Diagnosis of verrucous carcinoma in a biopsy or FS should be conservative and with great caution. Well-differentiated squamous cell carcinoma shows marked irregular infiltration, tumor necrosis, and prominent cytologic atypia (Figs. 3.15–3.18). Hyperplasia has similar morphological and cytologic features as those of verrucous carcinoma, but without deep tissue involvement and in some instances might be associated with development of verrucous carcinoma.

Warty carcinoma versus condyloma: Warty carcinoma is often large exophytic tumor with prominent HPV changes and prominent fibrovascular cores. The epithelial–stromal interface is infiltrative, pushing, or mixed. Helpful features to distinguish it from condyloma include larger size, more pronounced cytologic atypia, and infiltrative margin. Condyloma is often smaller, often with

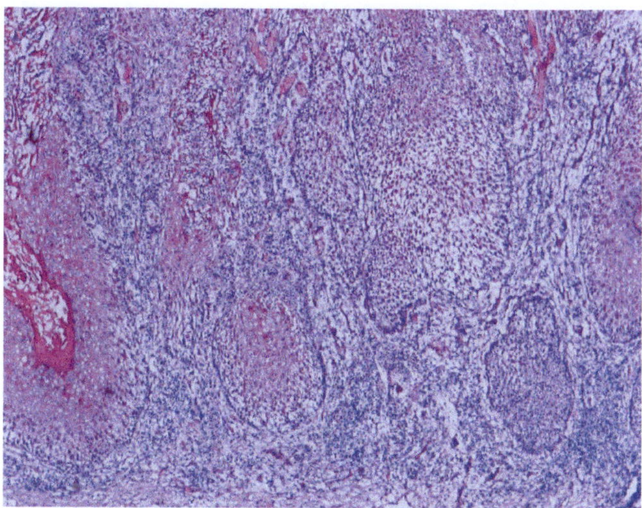

FIGURE 3.12 *Verrucous squamous cell carcinoma*. The tumor by definition is well differentiated. The tumor exhibits a characteristic broad-based "pushing" pattern of infiltration.

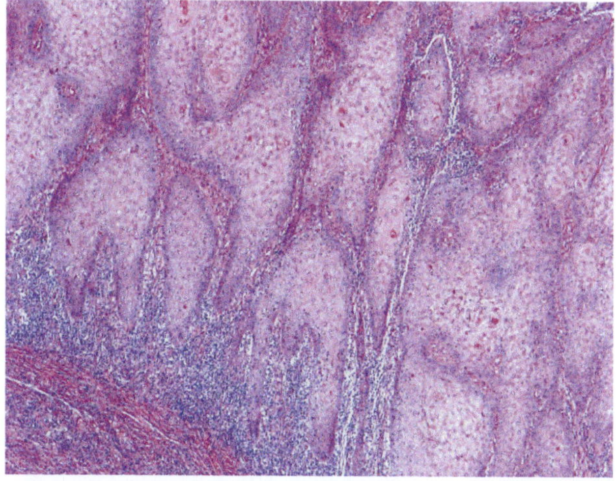

FIGURE 3.13 *Verrucous squamous cell carcinoma*. It is characterized by marked proliferation of tumor cells forming large nests with pushing margin toward the base. The tumor cells contain abundant eosinophilic to clear cytoplasm, low N/C ratio, and mild-to-moderate cytologic atypia. Chronic inflammation is evident at the interface with the deep fibroconnective tissue.

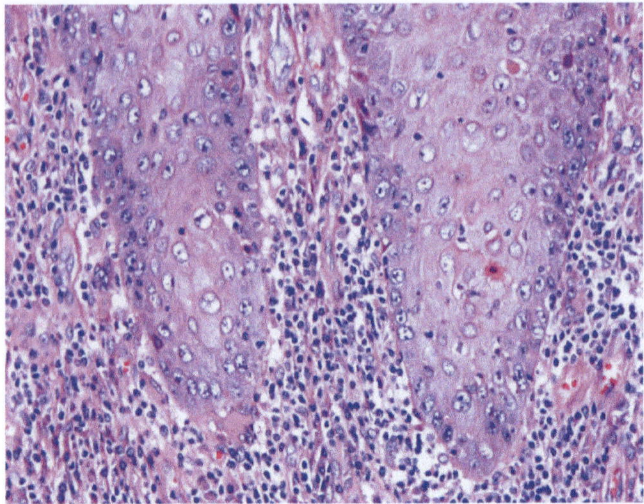

FIGURE 3.14 *Verrucous squamous cell carcinoma*. There is characteristic broad pushing margin with lack of destructive stromal invasion. The tumor cells are mild to moderately pleomorphic with rare mitoses. There is prominent chronic inflammation at the tumor base and stromal tissue.

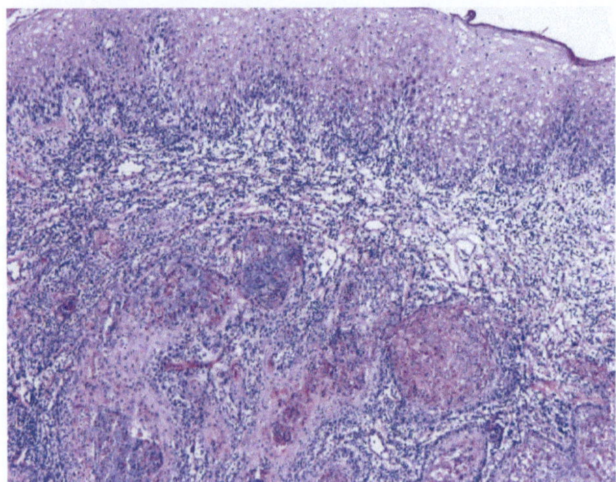

FIGURE 3.15 *Invasive well/moderately differentiated squamous cell carcinoma.* An invasive carcinoma with irregular infiltrating tumor cell nests with necrosis and keratinization. Extensive inflammation is present. The surface epithelium is uninvolved.

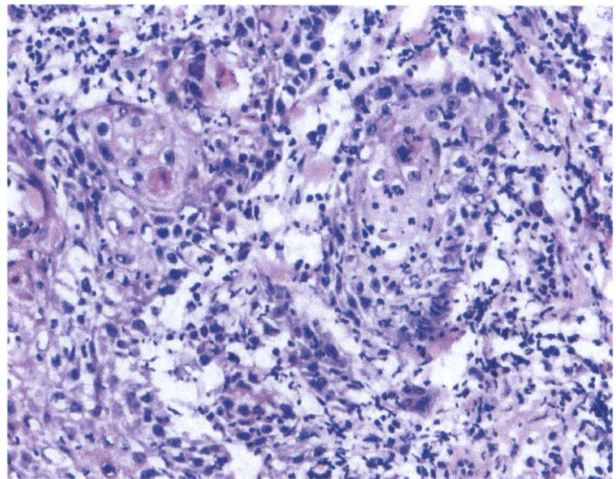

FIGURE 3.16 *Invasive squamous cell carcinoma*. The tumor is characterized by sheets or nests of tumor cells surrounded by desmoplastic stroma and chronic inflammation. Focal keratinization is present. Small clusters of single atypical cells are often helpful to make a definitive diagnosis of invasion.

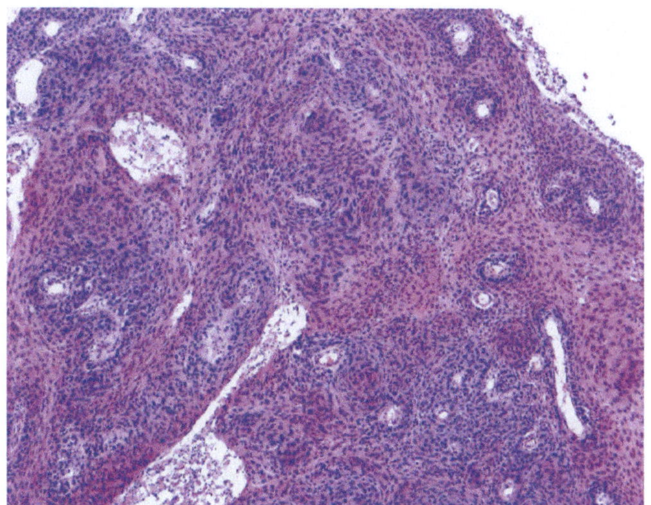

FIGURE 3.17 *Moderately differentiated squamous cell carcinoma*. A papillary squamous cell carcinoma with moderate cytologic atypia. Whether there is invasion cannot be evaluated.

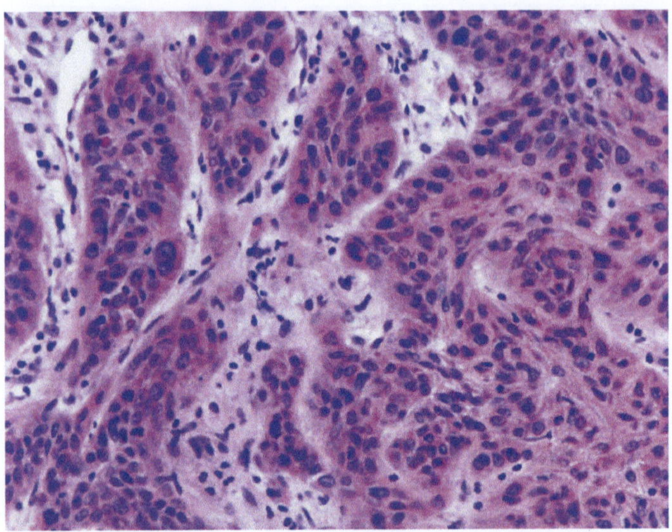

FIGURE 3.18 *Invasive moderately differentiated squamous cell carcinoma.* The tumor exhibits irregular nests of tumor cells with marked cytologic atypia and desmoplasia.

exuberant papillomatosis. Characteristic koilocytotic changes are usually evident and cytologic atypia is minimal (Fig. 3.19).

Sarcomatoid carcinoma versus pseudosarcomatous stromal reaction: Sarcomatoid carcinoma is most often associated with a better differentiated squamous cell carcinoma. Pseudoangiosarcomatous pattern can be prominent (Figs. 3.20–3.22). Multiple sections near or adjacent to the normal epithelium might be helpful for correct diagnosis. In situation of ulceration and florid chronic inflammation, granulation tissue or prior therapy, the diagnosis should be made with great caution.

Basal cell carcinoma versus basaloid squamous cell carcinoma: Basal cell carcinoma can occur in the penile skin (Figs. 3.23 and 3.24). It has the typical features as those of skin basal cell carcinoma occurring elsewhere. Basaloid squamous cell carcinoma, on the other hand, is often highly aggressive and deeply invasive. The tumor is composed of compact nests of basaloid tumor cells with high N/C ratio, inconspicuous nucleoli, and numerous mitotic features.

Seborrheic keratosis (SK) versus well-differentiated squamous cell carcinoma: SK is characterized by basaloid cell proliferation which can be papillomatous, resembling well-differentiated papillary squamous cell carcinoma. The differential features include lack of significant cytologic atypia, flat superficial lesion, and presence of horn cysts (Figs. 3.25 and 3.26).

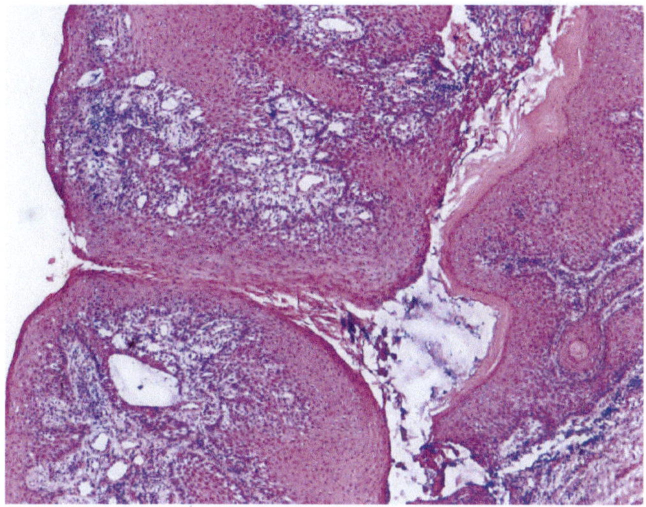

FIGURE 3.19 *Penile condyloma*. There is marked papillomatosis, hyperkeratosis, and acanthosis. Minimal cytologic atypia and koilocytotic changes are present.

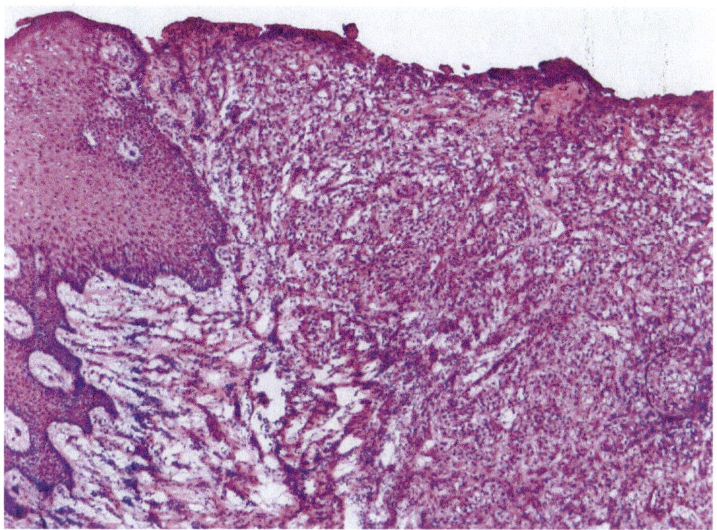

FIGURE 3.20 *Invasive squamous cell carcinoma with adjacent pseudoepitheliomatous hyperplasia.* The tumor is diffusely infiltrative with solid nests or cords of cells within a dense desmoplastic stroma.

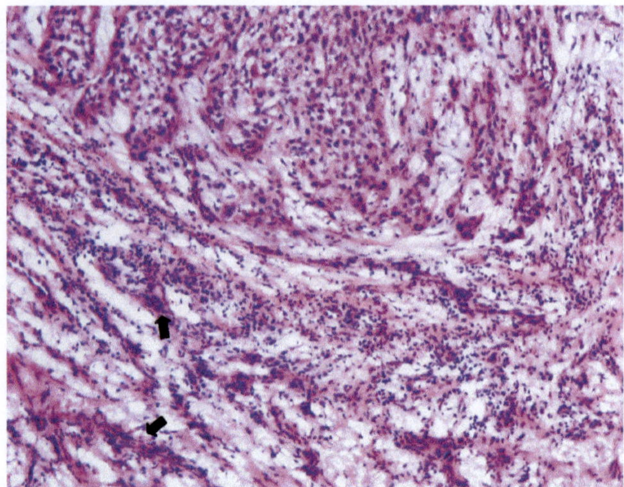

FIGURE 3.21 *Invasive squamous cell carcinoma.* The infiltrative tumor shows small clusters or cords of carcinomatous cells infiltrating the underlying fibroconnective tissue. There are also florid chronic inflammation and vascular proliferation (*arrows*), occasionally simulating invasive carcinoma on FS.

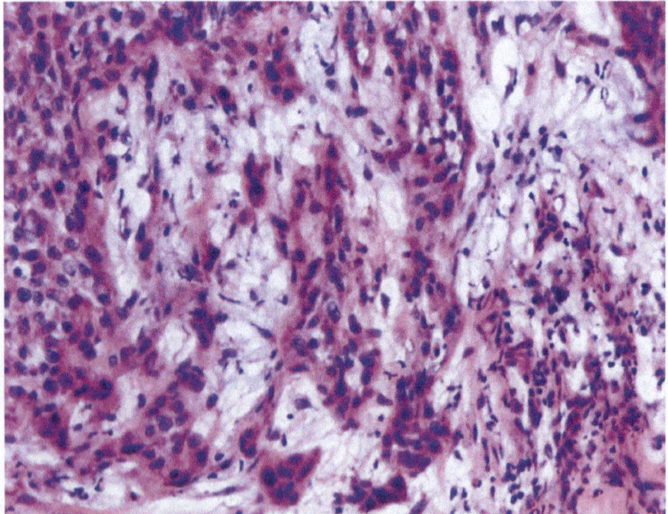

FIGURE 3.22 *Invasive squamous cell carcinoma.* The tumor shows irregular connecting cords (pseudovascular pattern) and chronic inflammation.

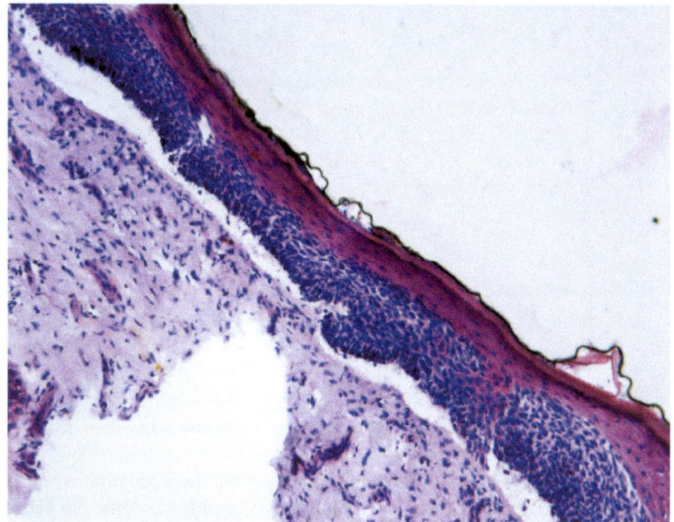

FIGURE 3.23 *Penile skin basal cell carcinoma of superficial type*. Proliferating basaloid cells at the base of the epidermis with characteristic pallisading and cleft around the tumor cells.

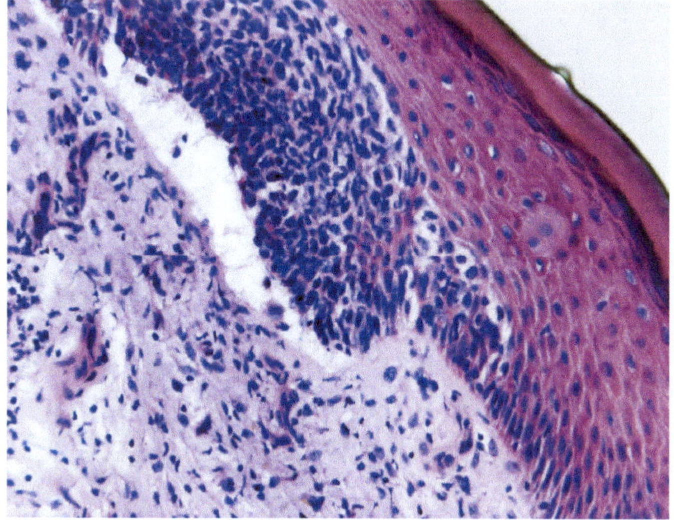

FIGURE 3.24 *Penile skin basal cell carcinoma of superficial type*. Proliferating basaloid cells at the base of the epidermis with characteristic pallisading and cleft around the tumor cells.

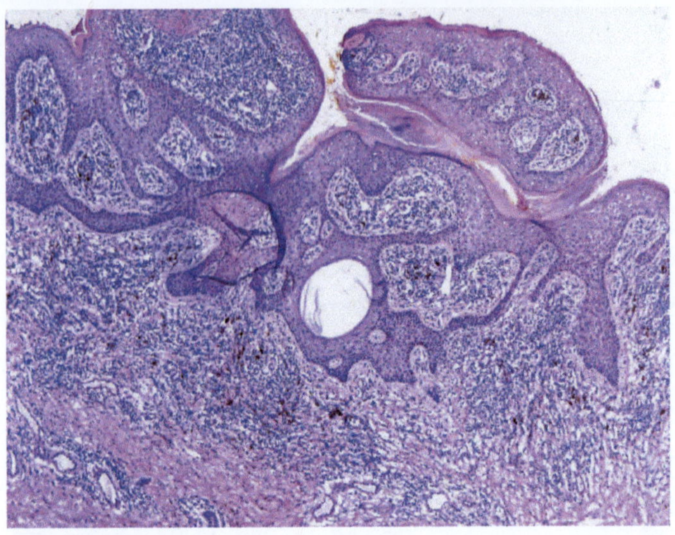

FIGURE 3.25 *Irritated seborrheic keratosis of penile skin.* There are proliferation of basaloid cells with a flat bottom, papillomatosis, and horn cysts. No significant cytologic atypia is present. Chronic inflammation is prominent.

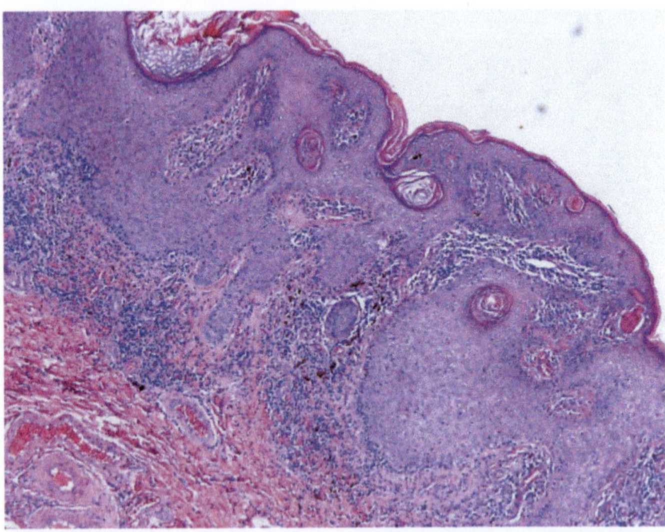

FIGURE 3.26 *Irritated seborrheic keratosis.* The lesion is characterized by marked proliferation of basaloid cells, papillomatosis, and horn cysts. No significant cytologic atypia is present. There are marked chronic inflammation and melanin pigment deposits.

EVALUATION OF LYMPH NODES DURING PENECTOMY

Clinical Background

Nodal metastasis remains the single most important prognostic factor for patients with penile cancer.[78] Approximately 20% of the patients with penile squamous cell carcinoma and clinically impalpable inguinal nodes at presentation will have occult micrometastasis.[79] Clinical examination and imaging techniques remain inaccurate for detecting micrometastasis. Superficial and modified inguinal nodal dissection techniques with intraoperative FS remain the "gold standard" for detecting the micrometastasis. In some centers, sentinel lymph node FS has shown to be effective in determining the extent of nodal dissection and therefore avoid unnecessary side effects of nodal dissection. In patients with well-differentiated squamous cell carcinoma and nonpalpable nodes, nodal dissection is not recommended. In patients with intermediate risk cancers (high grade and clinical T2) and without palpable nodes, sentinell lymph node biopsy with FS might be useful. In patients with poorly differentiated high-risk patients, nodal dissection with intraoperative FS is strongly recommended. Even in patients with palpable nodes, due to false positive findings of imaging and physical examination, FS is the only means to determine the extent of nodal dissection.

Specimen Handling

Sentinel or nonsentinel lymph nodes are carefully dissected from the fat tissue and all lymph node tissue should be submitted entirely for FS and avoid cutting too much tissue during the FS.

Interpretation

FS diagnosis of nodal metastasis of squamous cell carcinoma is often straightforward (Fig. 3.27). Cytologic imprint preparation can be a helpful adjunct for intraoperative FS diagnosis (Fig. 3.28).

For clinically negative nodal tissue, multiple levels might be cut to detect small focus of metastatic carcinoma. False negative diagnosis can result from small focus of metastatic basaloid or high grade squamous cell carcinoma, which can simulate germinal center of lymph node on FS. Occasionally confluent sinus histiocytosis or foamy macrophages can be erroneously interpreted as metastatic carcinoma.

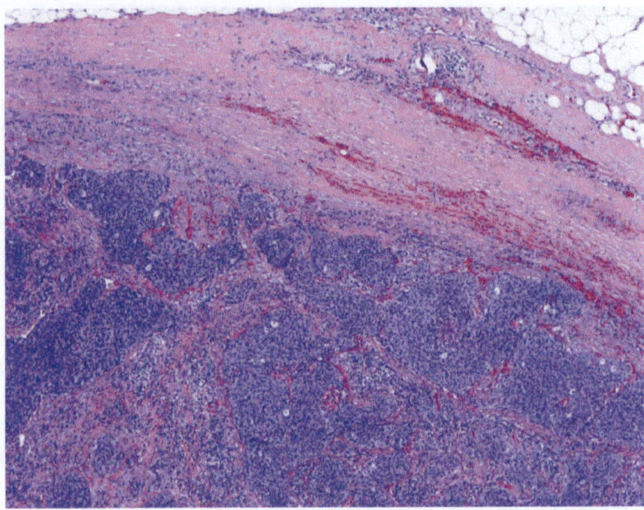

FIGURE 3.27 *Metastatic poorly differentiated squamous cell carcinoma*. Large sheets of basaloid tumor cells replace the lymph node and are surrounded by dense fibrotic capsule with obliteration of subcapsular sinuses.

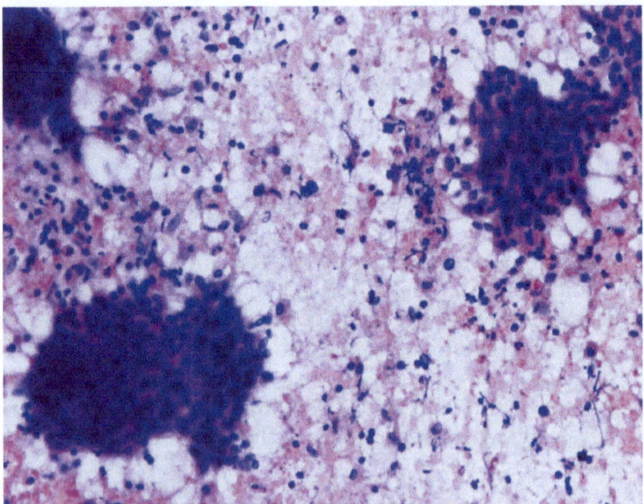

FIGURE 3.28 *Touch imprint cytology of a superficial inguinal lymph node showing metastatic poorly differentiated squamous cell carcinoma*. Nests of tumor cells with hyperchromatic and overlapping nuclei, and frequent apoptosis. The background shows tumor necrosis.

Chapter 4
Prostate

Ferran Algaba, Steven S. Shen, Luan D. Truong, and Jae Y. Ro

REASONS FOR INTRAOPERATIVE PATHOLOGY CONSULTATION

The widespread screening by measurement of serum prostatic specific antigen (PSA) and needle core biopsy allows more and more organ-confined prostate cancer being diagnosed. Orchiectomy as a treatment for prostate cancer almost completely disappears due to the availability of effective androgen ablative therapy. It is rarely necessary for the urologists to rely on intraoperative FS diagnosis for surgical treatment. However, there are still situations that FS is indicated for guidance of the surgical intervention as listed below:

1. Evaluation of surgical margin status during radical prostatectomy.
2. Evaluation of metastatic status of pelvic lymph nodes during radical prostatectomy.
3. Intraoperative diagnosis of adenocarcinoma in prostate from organ donors.
4. Intraoperative diagnosis of prostatic transurethral resection specimens, or simple prostatectomy specimens for nodular hyperplasia.

EVALUATION OF THE SURGICAL MARGINS

Clinical Background

The most common FS request in prostate cancer treatment is for the purpose of determining the status of the surgical margins during radical prostatectomy. In fact, the literature on the use and recommendation of FS for margin evaluation during radical prostatectomy is somewhat conflicting. Some investigators favor the routine use of FS as it may decrease the rate of final positive margins;[80,81] others argue against this practice.[82,83] Because of the

L.D. Truong et al., *Frozen Section Library: Genitourinary Tract,*
Frozen Section Library 2, DOI 10.1007/978-1-4419-0691-5_4,
© Springer Science + Business Media, LLC 2009

improved selection of patients eligible for radical prostatectomy, requests for intraoperative FS evaluation of margin status have decreased significantly. In most studies, positive margins at pathological examination have been shown to be associated with increased risk of biochemical disease recurrence. However, the clinical significance of a positive margin is still controversial. In one study, a significant proportion of patients with positive margins (65%) experience no biochemical failure.[84] This is the main reason for a lack of consensus on the use of FS.

In selective patients with high-risk disease, as determined by combination of clinical stage, Gleason score and PSA levels, FS can reliably predict the final surgical margin status when there are concerns about the margin status. Because of the relatively low predictive value of FS of the bladder neck and the neurovascular bundle/lateral pedicle, routine use of FS is not recommended. However, as more and more radical prostatectomy is performed for organ-confined early prostate cancer and in younger patients, preservation of neurovascular bundles and maintaining erectile function become critical. FS to determine whether they are affected by carcinoma will determine the feasibility of nerve-sparing surgery. Since it was shown that FS of the apex has a better predictive value for the final surgical margin,[83] most authors recommend FS of the apical margin to reduce the rate of final positive surgical margin and to maximize the urethral length, which should improve urinary continence of vesicourethral anastomosis.[82,85,86]

The area with the highest risk of positive surgical margin appears to depend at least in part on the surgical approach. Thus, the apex bears the highest risk in the retropubic approach, the bladder neck in the perineal approach, and the neurovascular bundles in the posterolateral aspect in the laparoscopic approach.[45] The latter observation and the fact that the neurovascular bundles are the main pathway for extraprostatic spread of tumor indicate that FS of the neurovascular bundles may be helpful when a laparoscopic nerve-sparing prostatectomy is performed with an attempt to preserve neurovascular bundles in patients with high risks for extraprostatic extension.

Specimen Handling

If biopsies from different surgical margins including the neurovascular bundle are submitted, the entire specimen should be submitted for FS evaluation. If evaluating margin status is requested on radical prostatectomy specimen, the urologist should indicate the suspicious areas by India ink or suture tie.[82] These areas should be repainted with permanent color ink (since India ink may not survive FS procedure), and perpendicular sections should be taken for FS to evaluate the margin status.

Interpretation

For intraoperative small biopsies submitted for FS, the presence of any neoplastic glands is considered a positive margin (Figs. 4.1–4.3). The diagnosis of prostatic carcinoma will rely on both architectural and cytologic features. The diagnostic criteria will be discussed in the following section. The presence of nonneoplastic glands should also be reported to the surgeon, as this finding may indicate inadequate removal of the prostate tissue or capsular incision.

For radical prostatectomy specimens, the interpretation and criteria used for FS margin evaluation should be identical to that for permanent sections. It is important to be aware of the artifacts associated with freezing and sampling. As most prostate cancer arising from the peripheral zone, for larger volume prostate cancers, the tumor tissue can come very close to the capsular margin. In order to make an unequivocal diagnosis of positive margin, the malignant glands have to come to direct contact with the inked margin. Evaluation of extraprostatic extension is usually not required during the intraoperative FS. For practical purposes, neoplastic glands in adipose tissue indicate extraprostatic extension (Fig. 4.4). Be cautious to report extraprostatic extension at FS as small amount of fat tissue can be seen within the prostatic parenchyma[87] and freezing artifact may simulate adipose tissue.

There are a number of pitfalls in interpretation of intraoperative FS. The causes of erroneous interpretations may include various artifacts (artifactual tear, crush, and thermal changes), anatomical variations (owing to lack of a true prostatic capsule),[88] the presence of intraprostatic fat,[87,89] and desmoplastic changes that are induced by invading carcinoma and mimic the periprostatic fibrous tissue.[90] In all of these situations, the diagnosis of extraprostatic extension and positive surgical margin should be made with great caution. Thermal artifact is particular problematic for interpretation of margin status and for distinction of benign from malignant glands. The constellation of multiple features including haphazard infiltrative pattern (Fig. 4.5), enlarged nuclei, prominent nucleoli, lack of basal cells (Fig. 4.6), and perineural invasion (Fig. 4.7) remains very helpful for a correct FS diagnosis. Cauterized nerves or ganglion tissue can simulate high-grade prostate carcinoma (Fig. 4.8). Similarly, small vessels with margination of neutrophils can also simulate carcinoma or lymphovascular invasion (Figs. 4.9 and 4.10). It is helpful to have recuts or deeper levels of those areas for a definitive diagnosis.

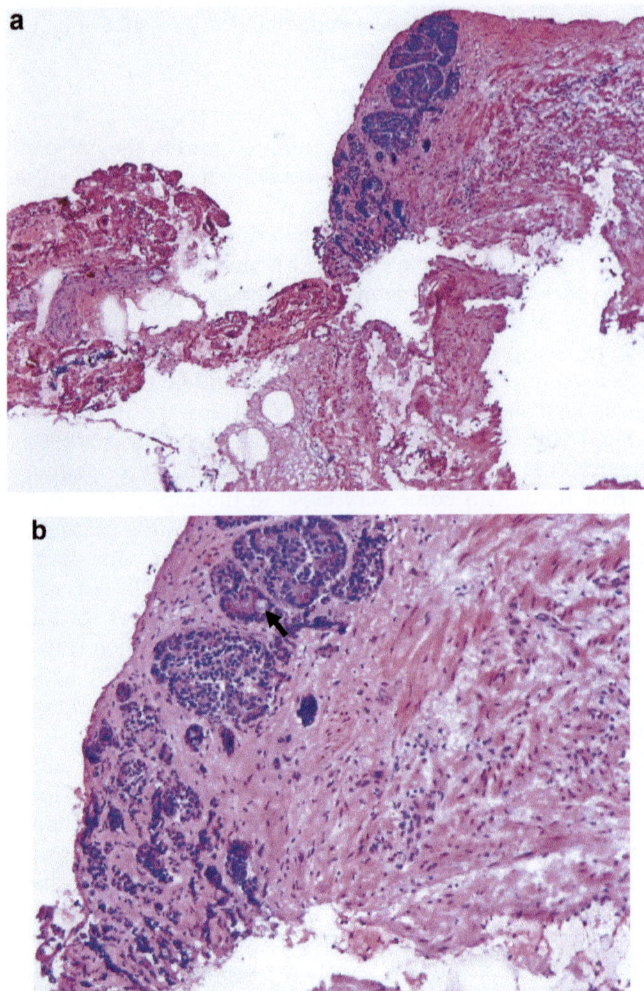

FIGURE 4.1. *FS of posterolateral margin biopsy.* (**a**) Low-power view shows the crowded small glands with fusion and irregular infiltrating edge, consistent with prostate carcinoma with a component of Gleason pattern 4 carcinoma. Notice also the freezing and cautery artifact on cancerous glands. Grading or assigning a Gleason score of tumor is not necessary. The presence of carcinoma indicates a positive margin. (**b**) Higher-power view shows prostate adenocarcinoma with cribriform and fused glands, focal intraluminal blue mucin (*arrow*) and irregular infiltrative growth.

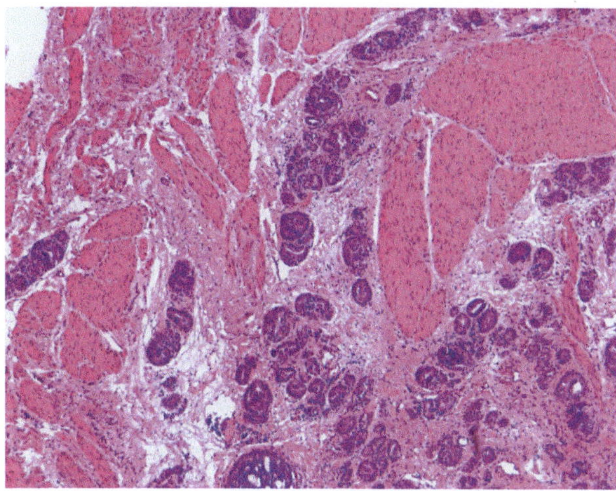

FIGURE 4.2. *Biopsy of bladder neck tissue with a positive margin*. Prostate carcinoma with haphazard infiltration of small neoplastic glands dissecting fibromuscular bundles of bladder neck. Large muscle bundles are typically seen in the biopsy from the bladder neck.

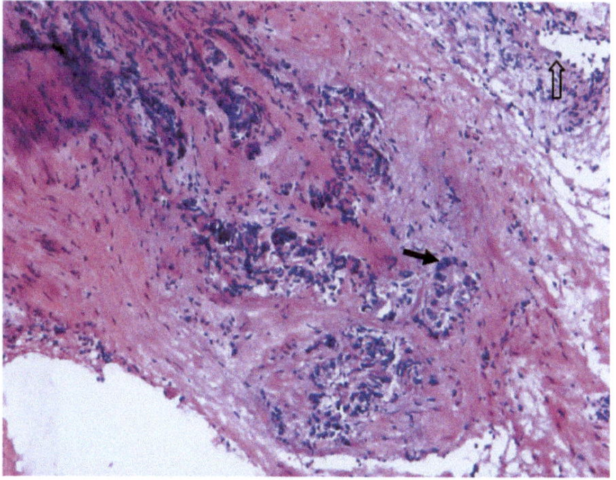

FIGURE 4.3. *Biopsy of apical tissue with positive margin*. There are crowded and fused glands infiltrating fibromuscular stroma. Although marked cautery artifacts are present, which obscure the cytologic details, the presence of markedly enlarge cells, nuclear pleomorphism, and prominent nucleoli, and lack of basal cells (*solid arrow*) are helpful features for the diagnosis of prostate carcinoma. The adjacent vascular endothelial cells (*open arrow*) and fibroblasts can serve as internal controls for the cell size.

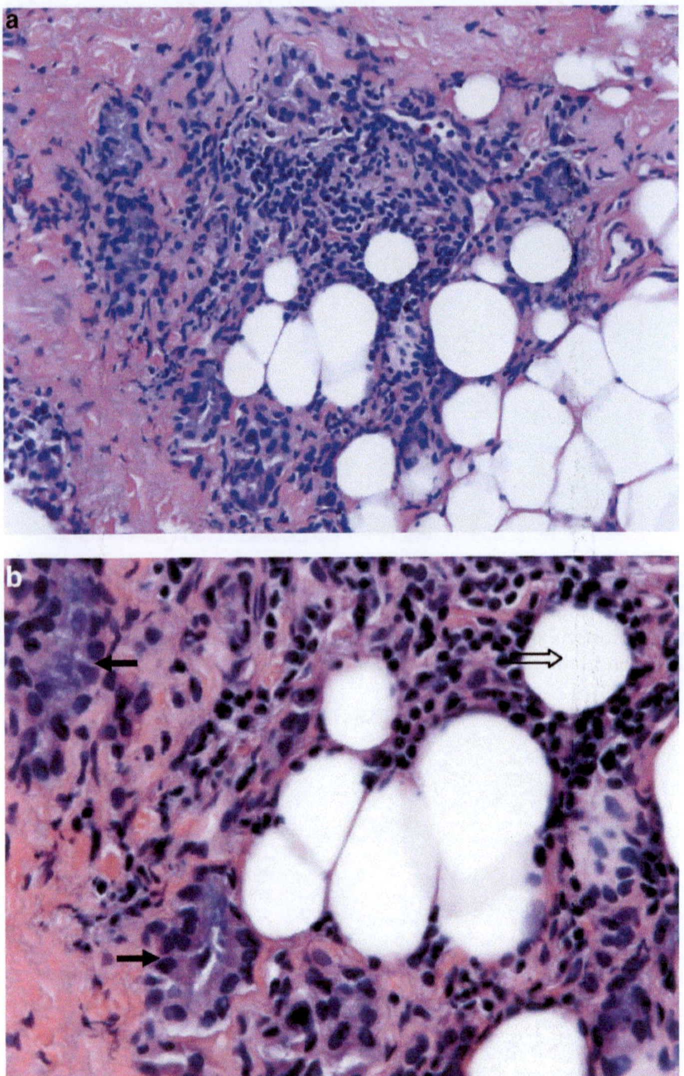

FIGURE 4.4. *Prostate carcinoma*. (**a**) Prostate carcinoma with neoplastic glands within the adipose tissue and also chronic inflammation. Although intraparenchymal adipose tissue has been reported in the prostate, the presence of fat tissue admixed with glandular components (abnormal location) is highly consistent with extraprostatic extension of carcinoma. (**b**) Infiltrating prostate carcinoma with neoplastic glands that are difficult to identify on FS. Small glands with a single layer for the lining cells, occasional nucleoli, and rigid lumen are helpful features of diagnosis of carcinoma (*solid arrows*). Lymphocytic infiltration can obscure the glandular architecture and can appear as pseudogland (*open arrow*) surrounded by lymphocytes.

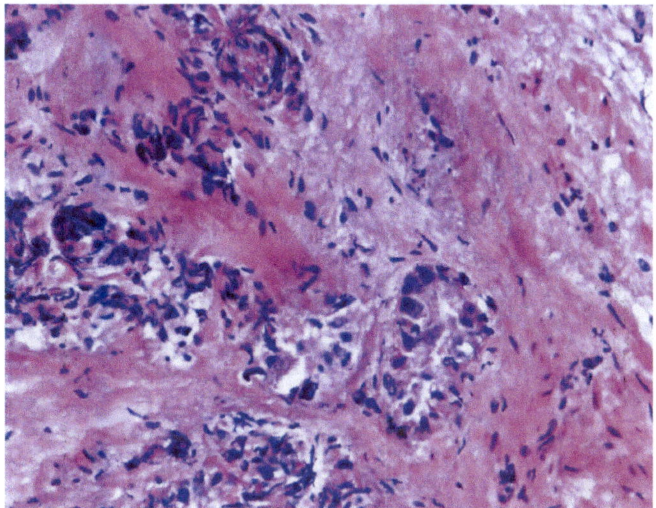

FIGURE 4.5. *Biopsy of lateral surgical margin with carcinoma*. An irregular infiltrative and haphazard growth pattern is helpful diagnostic features of carcinoma in spite of marked cautery artifact.

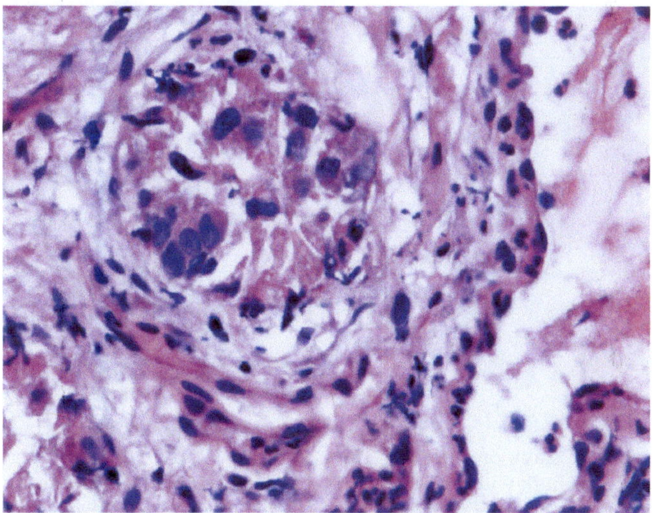

FIGURE 4.6. *Biopsy of apical margin*. High-power view shows one atypical gland with large nuclei and prominent nucleoli, highly suspicious for adenocarcinoma. Lack of basal cells and dense amphophilic cytoplasm are also helpful for the diagnosis of carcinoma.

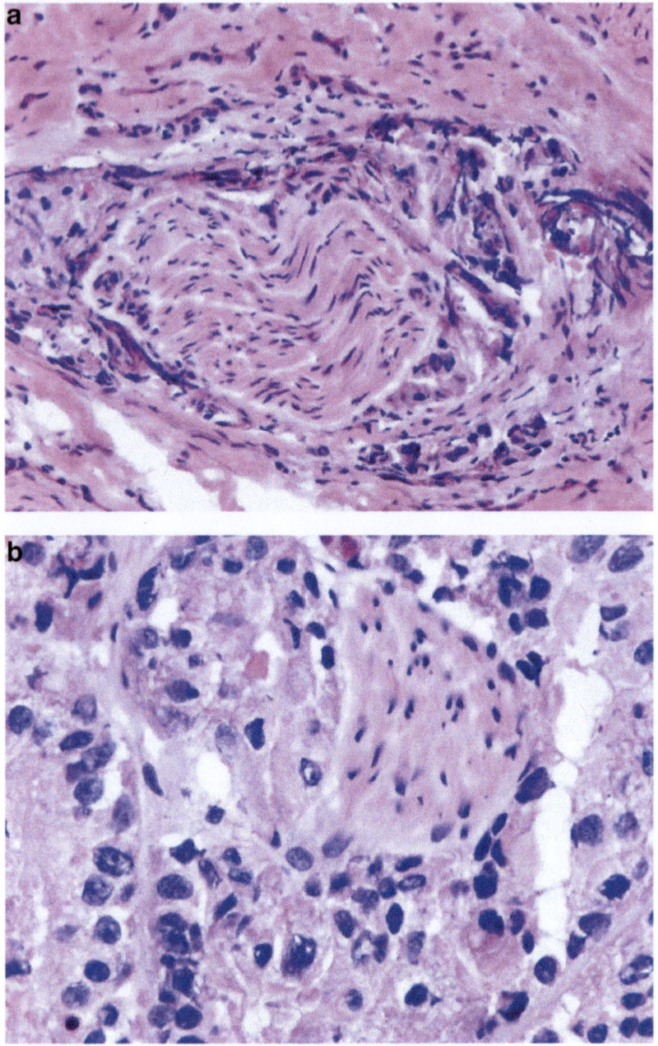

FIGURE 4.7. *Biopsy of posterolateral margin.* (**a**) Circumferential perineural invasion by carcinoma glands. There is marked cautery artifact of glandular epithelium with nuclear debris with condensation around the nerve tissue. In spite of poor cytologic detail, perineural invasion is diagnostic for carcinoma. (**b**) High-power view of neoplastic glands with circumferential perineural invasion. The tumor cells show large nuclei and prominent nucleoli. Identification of nerve fibers and their relationship with epithelial component is helpful for the diagnosis.

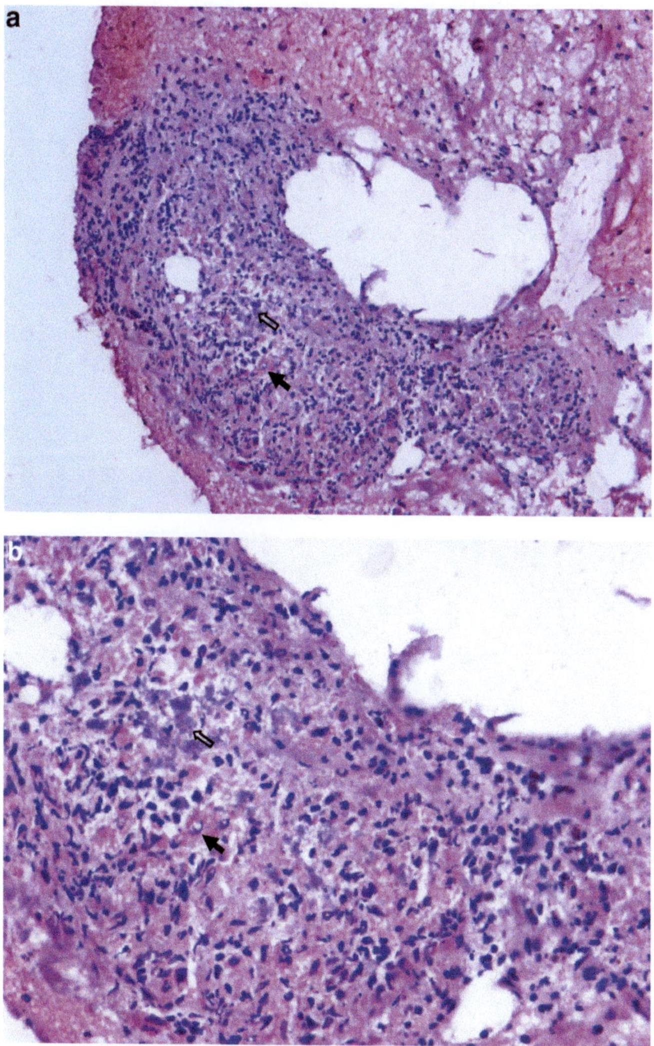

FIGURE 4.8. *Ganglion cells and nerve simulating carcinoma.* (**a**) Cauterized ganglion cells and nerve can resemble poorly differentiated cribriform prostate carcinoma. They are often well circumscribed with evenly distributed cellular elements with large ganglion cells (*solid arrow*) with prominent basophilic granular cytoplasm (*open arrow*). Ganglion cells may not be evident. (**b**) High-power view of the same field.

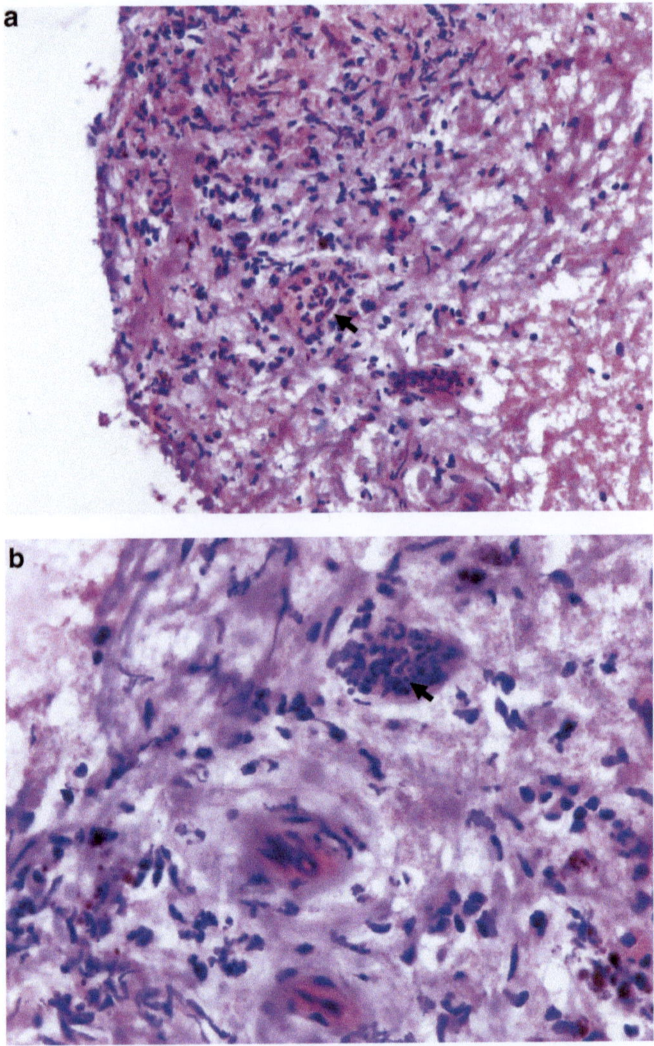

FIGURE 4.9. *Blood vessels simulating carcinoma.* (**a**) Inflammatory cells and vessels filled with neutrophils mimicking prostate cancer (*arrow*) when associated with marked freezing and cautery artifact. (**b**) Arteries and veins with intravascular margination of white blood cells resembling glandular elements.

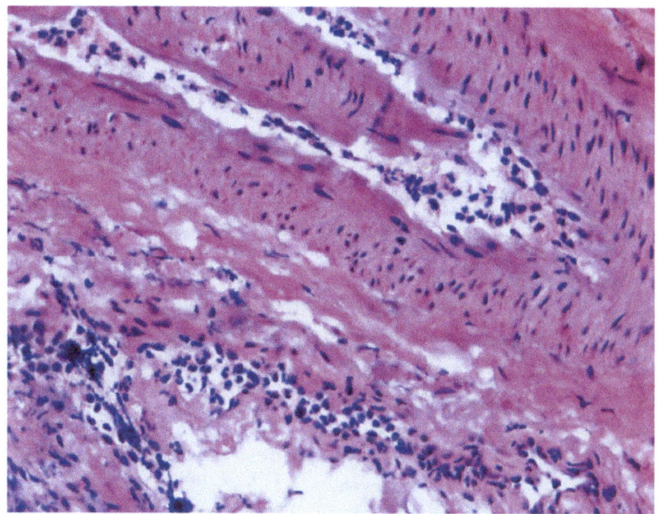

FIGURE 4.10. *Inflammatory cells simulating carcinoma.* Margination of neutrophils within large thick-walled arteries and veins may mimic vascular invasion or prostate carcinoma.

If a definitive diagnosis still cannot be reached after deeper sections, another biopsy for FS may be requested or the definitive diagnosis is deferred to permanent sections.

EVALUATION OF PELVIC LYMPH NODES DURING RADICAL PROSTATECTOMY

Clinical Background

Lymph node dissection is an integral part of TNM staging and is potentially therapeutic, when performed with radical prostatectomy. Furthermore, nodal metastasis implies disseminated carcinoma and is generally a contraindication of radical prostatectomy as a treatment for prostatic carcinoma. With more and more early and localized prostate cancer being treated by radical prostatectomy, there is an apparent stage migration in recent years. Routine FS of the lymph nodes during radical prostatectomy may not be necessary for all patients. First, the incidence of nodal metastasis in radical prostatectomy continues to decrease from 5.2–7.9% in some previous series to 1–2% recently. This reduced incidence is most likely due to serum PSA screening with early cancer detection and also due to better case selection on clinical criteria.

Furthermore, a number of nomograms based on serum PSA, biopsy Gleason score, and clinical tumor stage and others have been developed to predict the risk of lymph node metastasis.[91] Thus, in patients with a low or intermediate risk, the chance of nodal metastasis is minimal and therefore FS may not be needed.[92] However, for patients with high risk of nodal metastasis, positive nodal metastasis by FS may help the surgeon to decide on aborting or proceeding with radical prostatectomy.[93]

Specimen Handling

The choice of FS versus gross examination will be determined by urologists and pathologists together based on clinical and gross findings. Some have suggested that all lymph nodes should be submitted for FS in cases with a Gleason score of 8 or higher.[94] If the Gleason score is lower than 8, gross evaluation alone or examination of two or three representative nodes (selected on the basis of size and consistency) is recommended.[95]

All lymph nodes should be serially sectioned in 3–4 mm intervals and carefully examined grossly. For patients with low risk of nodal metastasis, gross examination might be sufficient. However, any areas that are suspicious for metastatic carcinoma grossly should be submitted for FS.

Interpretation

The specificity of FS diagnosis of nodal metastasis approaches 100%. The sensitivity reaches 100% if there are grossly suspicious lesions but much lower (67%) in cases of micrometastasis with a false negative rate of 33%.[92,96] These data suggest that if FS is to be performed on a grossly negative lymph node, serial slices of the entire lymph node should be submitted to FS.

Metastatic high-grade metastatic carcinoma with cribriform gland formation or comedo-type necrosis is relatively easy to diagnose by FS. High-grade carcinoma tends to induce desmoplastic reaction, which facilitates its recognition in FS (Fig. 4.11). However, well-differentiated tumors often lack desmoplasia and their cytologic features are relatively bland (Figs. 4.12 and 4.13). Small focus of metastasis, particularly when they are subjected to freezing artifact, can easily be overlooked. Metastatic high-grade Gleason pattern 5 carcinoma and tumors composed of signet ring cells or foamy cells can simulate and misinterpreted as sinus histiocytes. Conversely, false positive FS result has been reported in patients with hip joint replacement, in whom the pelvic lymph nodes may be extensively infiltrated with foamy histiocytes and they can closely simulate metastatic prostate cancer cells[97] (Fig. 4.14). Similar to other locations, reactive intranodal vascular

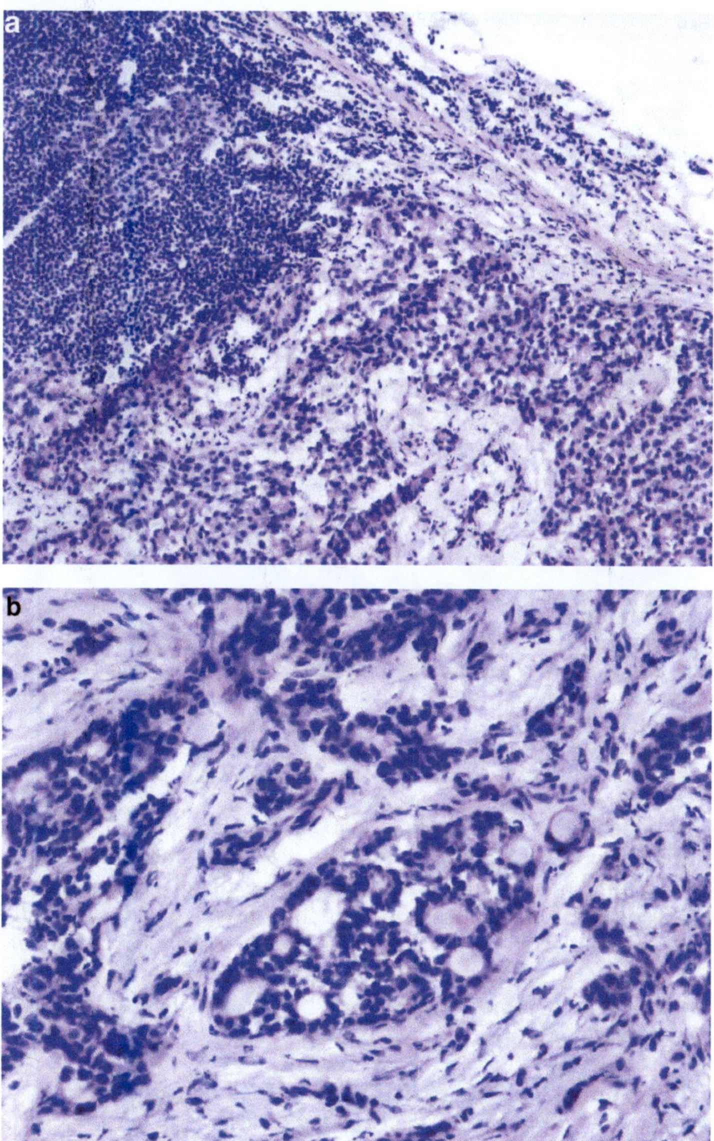

FIGURE 4.11. *Metastatic prostate carcinoma to lymph node*. (a) high-grade carcinoma with diffuse sheets of neoplastic glands, poorly formed glandular lumens, and surrounding desmoplastic stroma. (**b**) High-grade carcinoma with cribriform glands and abundant desmoplastic reaction. Different from many other types of carcinoma, prostate cancerous glands typically are composed of relatively monotonous tumor cells with no significant pleomorphism.

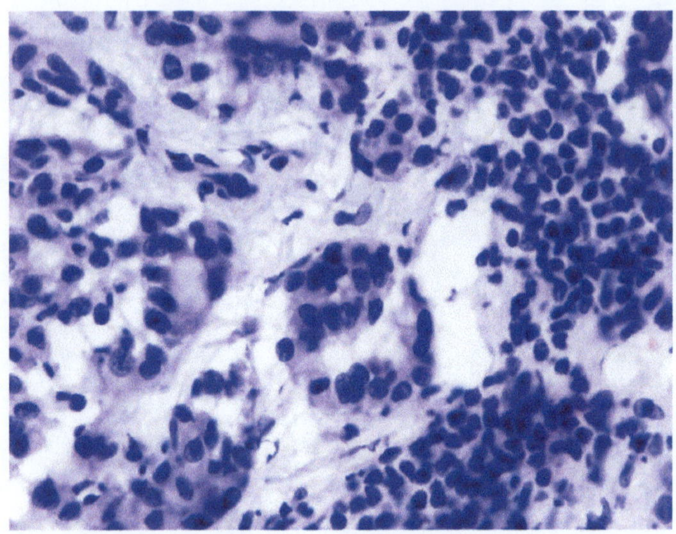

FIGURE 4.12. *Metastatic prostatic acinar adenocarcinoma to lymph node.* The tumor cells have uniformly enlarged nuclei, regular nuclear membrane, and prominent nucleoli. There is minimal or no desmoplastic reaction.

spaces can mimic metastatic adenocarcinoma as well (Fig. 4.15). Rarely, sinus histiocytes can have a signet ring appearance, particularly on FS, and can lead to false positive diagnosis of metastatic carcinoma. Intranodal inclusion-type glands with cells showing Mullerian features have also been rarely reported in pelvic lymph nodes in men.[98] Awareness of these pitfalls and review the previous biopsy material before FS are very helpful for a correct interpretation.

FROZEN SECTION DIAGNOSIS OF ADENOCARCINOMA IN PROSTATES FROM ORGAN DONORS

Clinical Background

Organ transplantation has been increasingly performed in recent years. Both organ recipients and donors may harbor a clinically silent, but significant prostate cancer. Many types of solid cancer can occur in patients after transplantation including very rarely prostate adenocarcinoma. So far only one documented case of prostate carcinoma was developed in a patient of heart recipient.[99] FS is usually not requested for the purpose of detecting occult prostate

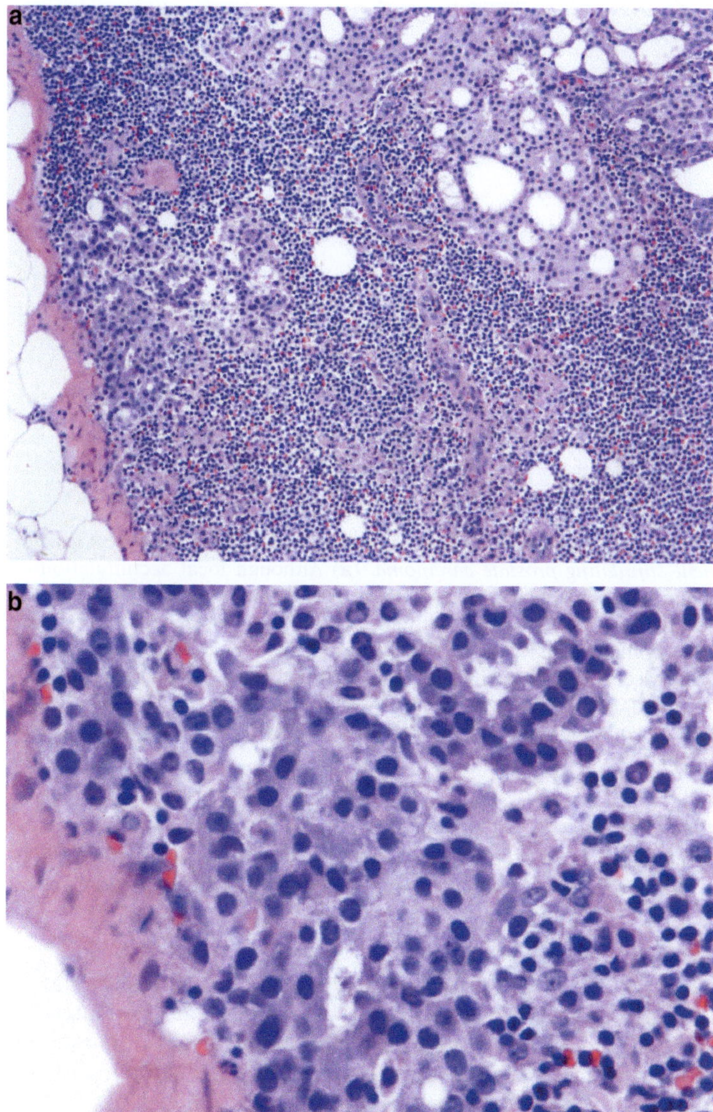

FIGURE 4.13. *Metastatic prostatic acinar adenocarcinoma to lymph node.* (**a**) Tumor tissue with acini and glands with relatively small nuclei and minimal desmoplasia. These glands are still relatively cohesive with sharp demarcation from lymphoid cells. (**b**) The tumor cells have relatively bland cytologic features with small nuclei, round to ovoid nuclei, homogenous chromatin, and small nucleoli.

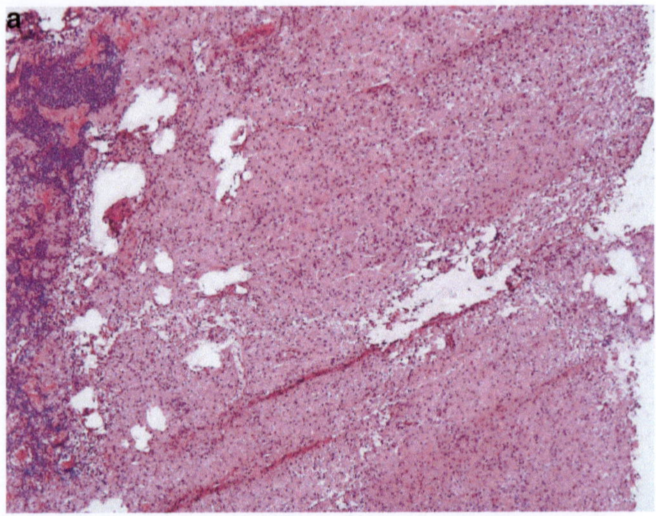

FIGURE 4.14. *Accumulation of histiocytes in lymph node due to joint replacement simulating prostate carcinoma.* (a) Although focal accumulation of macrophages/histiocytes is frequent in pelvic lymph node, the type of histiocytic reaction associated with knee or hip joint replacement, as shown here, is characteristic for this condition, if this type of lesion is aware of. Otherwise, it can be easily confused with metastatic high-grade prostatic carcinoma. It is characterized by extensive replacement of pelvic lymph node by contiguous, closely packed histiocytes without desmoplastic stromal reaction.

carcinoma. However, if the donor have a high-serum PSA, it is important to rule out the possibility of significant prostate cancer.

Specimen Handling

It is impractical to do FS of entire prostate. The prostate should be sectioned transversely from apex to bladder neck at 3 mm intervals and examined carefully with suspicious areas being submitted for FS. If suspicious lesions are not seen, extensive sampling of the peripheral zone will be the important as the majority of prostate cancer arise from this zone. If this procedure does not disclose a carcinoma, it is generally accepted that the donor is free of prostate carcinoma.[100]

Interpretation

See in following section.

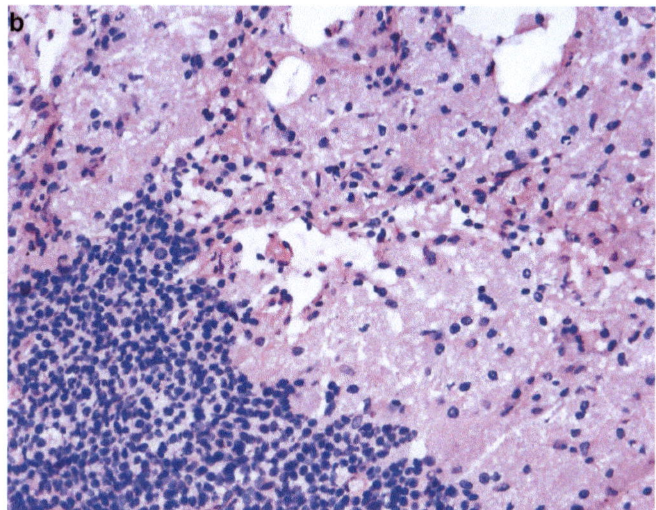

FIGURE 4.14. (**b**) On higher magnification, these histiocytes are characterized by cells with very abundant foamy cytoplasm, small round to ovoid nuclei. There is no discernible gland formation or nested pattern of carcinoma. The N/C ratio is much higher and the nuclei are smaller than that of prostate carcinoma.

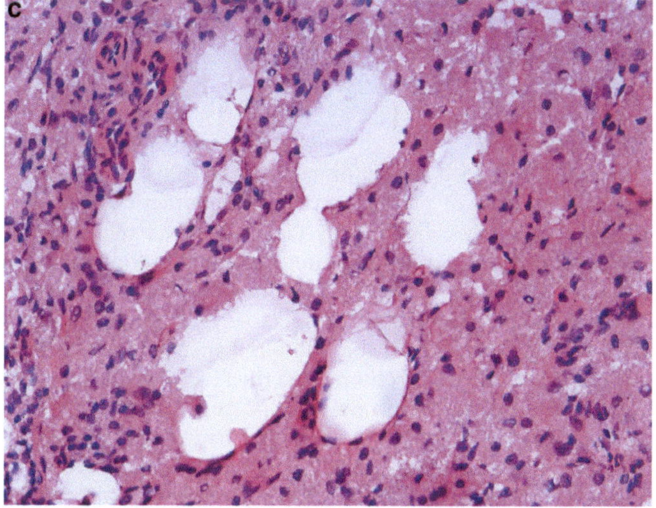

FIGURE 4.14. (**c**) Replacement of pelvic lymph node by foamy histiocytes resembling high-grade or foamy gland metastatic adenocarcinoma. Freezing artifact can simulate glands.

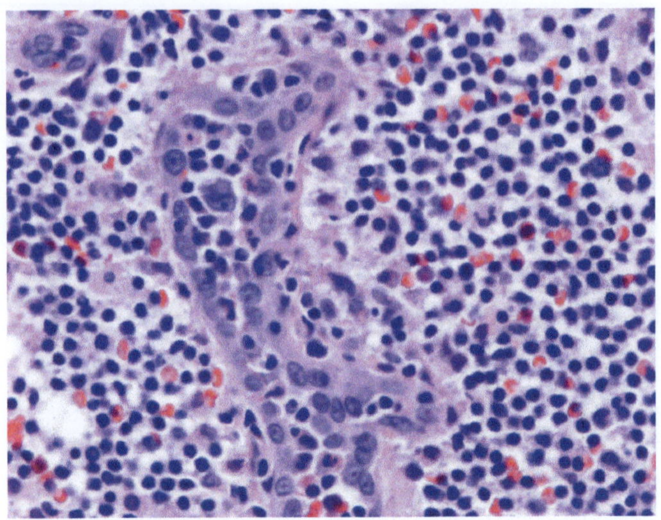

FIGURE 4.15. *Reactive intranodal postcapillary venules*. The blood vessel shows plump endothelial cells with prominent nucleoli, which may mimic carcinomatous glands.

FROZEN SECTION DIAGNOSIS OF ADENOCARCINOMA IN PROSTATIC TRANSURETHRAL RESECTION SPECIMENS, OR SIMPLE PROSTATECTOMY SPECIMENS FOR NODULAR HYPERPLASIA

Clinical Background

In the past, FS of core needle biopsy had been used for the intra-operative diagnosis of prostate cancer. This practice is no longer acceptable as preoperative biopsy diagnosis is an integral part of risk assessment and surgery planning. More importantly, the reliability of FS in this context is rather poor.[101] In some institutions, transurethrally resected prostate specimens or simple prostatectomy specimens performed for nodular hyperplasia may be submitted for FS to detect carcinoma. In the past, this has been done mainly for the purpose of immediate postoperative patient counseling. However, this practice should be strongly discouraged due to frequent false positive or false negative results associated with sampling or FS artifacts. Even when the diagnosis of carcinoma is correctly made, grading, especially for the low-grade tumors, is extremely unreliable. In addition, the diagnosis of carcinoma rarely changes the course of surgery.

Specimen Handling

For transurethrally resected prostate specimens, the amount of tissue selected for FS is not well defined. In one study, selecting areas with a firmer than normal consistency and a yellowish hue affords a 100% specificity and a 39% sensitivity in diagnosing prostate cancer.[102] In simple prostatectomy specimen, sampling of the indurate area in the peripheral zones of the prostate has the best chance to identify carcinoma.

Interpretation: Diagnosis of Well Differentiated Prostate Carcinoma

The diagnosis of prostate cancer relies on the architectural and cytology features. Similar to permanent tissue section, prostate cancer diagnosis is based on a number of criteria, the most important of which are the architecture of gland proliferation (small glands, cribriform growths, and solid and cord masses), nuclear atypia with large nucleoli, and absence of basal cells.[103] At low power, when the glands are too small and too crowded, and the glandular cell cytoplasm is too clear, it should be further evaluated at high power for helpful diagnostic features including enlarged nuclei, prominent nucleoli, and lack of basal cells.[104] The absence of basal cells may be very difficult to evaluated in intraoperative FS, as it may only be demonstrated with immunohistochemical methods.[105] Although rapid immunohistochemical methods are being developed, these are not yet implemented or practical in routine FS practice. One very useful diagnostic feature for carcinoma is the demonstration of circumferential perineural invasion. But be aware of the fact that benign or atrophic glands may abut nerves.

Although the majority of the prostate carcinomas are micro-acinar with proliferation of well-formed small glands, high-grade carcinoma may show cribriform or solid growth patterns or single cells. It must be noted, however, that there are multiple benign morphologic mimickers of prostatic adenocarcinoma.[106-109] It is often difficult to recognize them on FS. The most common entities and their salient diagnostic features are summarized here:

Sclerosing adenosis: In one study, this condition accounts for some 25% of the diagnostic errors.[43] The features that are helpful to distinguish it from an adenocarcinoma are greater variation of the gland size and shape, the thickened basement membrane, and the cellular stroma composed of myoepithelial cells.[110]

Atypical adenomatous hyperplasia: This lesion, also called prostatic adenosis,[109] is also a common benign mimicker of well-differentiated carcinoma.[43,111,112] It is considered to be a precursor lesion of transition zone prostate carcinoma, although this is still not well established. At low-power magnification, *atypical adenomatous hyperplasia* has a similar microglandular growth pattern as that of well-differentiated prostate carcinoma. The key distinguishing features are that the cells lack of prominent nucleoli and the gland retains basal cells, at least partially.

Basal cell hyperplasia: This lesion is commonly found within the context of benign prostatic hyperplasia in transition zone, but it can occur in the peripheral zone as well.[113] Helpful diagnostic features for basal cell hyperplasia include multiple cell layers, cytoplasmic basophilia, and absence of prominent nucleoli. The so-called atypical basal cell hyperplasia may be mistaken for prostatic carcinoma because it often exhibit prominent nucleoli and cytologic atypia.[113]

Prostate atrophy: This is a very common and morphologically variable lesion. It accounts for most of the erroneous diagnoses of adenocarcinoma at the peripheral area of the prostate in core needle biopsies.[111,112] The most useful diagnostic feature for atrophy is the preservation of lobular architecture of glandular units at low-power magnification. Prostatic atrophy also lacks prominent nucleoli and basal cells are partially maintained. It is important to note that prostate carcinoma with a pseudoatrophic pattern can also rarely occur.[114] FS diagnosis in this situation can be particularly treacherous.

Clear cell cribriform hyperplasia: Prostatic nodular hyperplasia may adopt focally cribriform and clear cell appearance that is likely to be mistaken for high-grade prostate adenocarcinoma. Basal cells are preserved and even focally hyperplastic in this lesion and the component cells lack prominent nucleoli.[109]

Reactive atypia associated with inflammation or treatment: Glandular reactive atypia secondary to either inflammation or previous hormonal or radiation therapy may be extremely difficult to diagnose.[115] In these situations, careful assessment of the architectural pattern and clinical correlation are essential for avoidance of an incorrect diagnosis.[109]

Nephrogenic adenoma: It has a variety of growth patterns including microglandular structures or acini, similar to that of prostate carcinoma. However, it occurs almost exclusively in periurethral location and often has smaller acini than those in prostate carcinoma.[116,117] Because nephrogenic adenoma is frequently negative for basal cell markers and positive for racemase (P504S), immunohistochemical results can further complicate the distinction. In this situation, immunostain for PSA or prostatic acid phosphatase should be helpful to exclude their prostatic gland origin.

Other benign mimickers of prostate cancer: Other small gland mimickers of prostate cancer include mesonephric hyperplasia, mucinous metaplasia, and verumontanum mucosal gland hyperplasia, and normal anatomic structures such as Cowper's glands, seminal vesicle, or ejaculatory duct.[43]

Diagnosis of High-Grade Prostatic Carcinoma

Benign conditions that may mimic high-grade prostate carcinoma: These include xanthogranulomatous inflammation, malakoplakia, granulomatous prostatitis, transitional and squamous metaplasia induced by inflammation or previous procedures, and rarely normal paraganglia. The main features that differentiate high-grade prostate carcinoma from benign conditions are their cytological findings including uniform nuclear enlargement and prominent nucleoli.

Malignant neoplasms that may mimic high-grade prostate carcinoma: These include prostatic urothelial carcinoma, colorectal cancers, and metastatic cancers from other sites. Helpful features including relatively monotonous nuclei, prominent nucleolus, and lower number of mitoses favor high-grade prostate carcinoma. In contrast, marked nuclear pleomorphism, variable nucleolar prominence, and frequent mitoses favor nonprostatic malignancy.[104]

Chapter 5
Testis

Ferran Algaba, Ja e Y.Ro , St even S. Shen,
andL uan D. Truong

REASONS FOR INTRAOPERATIVE CONSULTATION

Intraoperative consultation including FS of testicular lesions is infrequently performed, since the available diagnostic imaging techniques and serum tumor markers permit most neoplasia to be diagnosed prior to orchiectomy. However, the number of cases of conservative surgical management is increasing in which the urologist performs an intraoperative analysis of the testicular lesion in order to be able to perform testis-sparing surgery. The possible reasons for intraoperative consultation are listed in Table 5.1

GROSS CONSULTATION ON RADICAL ORCHIECTOMY SPECIMEN

Clinical Background

The vast majority of testicular tumors are germ cell neoplasia diagnosed preoperatively by clinical and imaging findings. They are treated by radical orchiectomy through the inguinal approach since the scrotal approach may cause tumor tissue contamination of the scrotal skin, which alters the pattern of potential nodal metastasis. The specimen may be submitted for intraoperative gross consultation to evaluate the surgical margins and documentation of a gross tumor mass. FS of the tumor is often not requested since the diagnosis would not alter intraoperative treatment. Furthermore, in many nonneoplastic conditions, the lesion may be very extensive and completely destroys the testicular parenchyma. That is why organ preservation is not considered and, therefore, FS evaluation is usually not needed.

L.D. Truong et al., *Frozen Section Library: Genitourinary Tract*,
Frozen Section Library 2, DOI 10.1007/978-1-4419-0691-5_5,
© Springer Science + Business Media, LLC 2009

TABLE 5.1 Reasons for intraoperative consultation for testicular lesions.

Gross consultation on radical orchiectomy specimen
    To evaluate surgical margins
    To confirm the presence of a testicular tumor
Frozen section consultation for partial orchiectomy
    Tumor mass in prepubertal patients
    Nonpalpable asymptomatic incidental mass
    Mass suspicious to be benign neoplasms or of nonneoplastic natures
    Synchronous bilateral germ cell tumors or unilateral germ cell tumor
      with a history of contralateral orchiectomy for germ cell tumor
Gross consultation/frozen section of lymph node in retroperitoneal
    nodal dissection
Frozen section/touch preparation of testicular biopsy for infertility
Touch preparation in vasectomy reversal

Specimen Handling

The radical orchiectomy specimen consists of the testis, the surrounding tunica vaginalis which is separated from the testis by a potential space, the epididymis, and a portion of the spermatic cord. The tunica vaginalis is composed a single layer of mesothelial cells resting on the internal spermatic fascia, which is composed of connective tissue loosely attached to the scrotal wall. This loose attachment permits removal of the radical orchiectomy specimen by mechanical pulling of the spermatic cord through the inguinal canal.

The surgical margin is the entire outer surface of the tunica vaginalis and the end of the spermatic cord. Since the tunica albuginea surrounding the testis is very resistant to tumor spread, tumor extension through the tunica albuginea to involve the tunica vaginalis surgical margin is extremely rare. The outer surface of tunica vaginalis is examined for tumor involvement and cut open to expose the testis. The testis is examined and bisected through a sagittal plane to expose the cut surface of the testis, the testicular mediastinum, and the epididymis. This should allow recognition of the lesion and its relationship to the surrounding structures including the surgical margins, but additional sections parallel or perpendicular to the original plane may be needed.

Interpretation

The status of the surgical margins should be obvious by gross examination. If gross findings are equivocal, tissue may be submitted for FS, noting that contamination of these tissue samples by the blades already used to section the tumor often occurs, and this should be prevented by using a new blade or taking the surgical margin before sectioning the tumor. We recommend taking surgical margin first before opening the testis. Even when FS diagnosis of the lesion is not requested, it may be performed at the discretion of the pathologist in selected cases depending on the gross and clinical features, since a specific diagnosis may permit allocation of fresh tissue for special studies (e.g., flow cytometry for lymphoma, cultures for infectious organisms, or cytogenetic profiling).

FROZEN SECTION CONSULTATION FOR A SPECIFIC DIAGNOSIS PRIOR TO SURGERY FOR POSSIBLE TESTIS-SPARING OPERATION

Clinical Background

Radical orchiectomy without FS consultation is the standard treatment for germ cell tumor. Even when the germ cell tumor is small, testis-sparing partial orchiectomy is not indicated (Fig. 5.1),

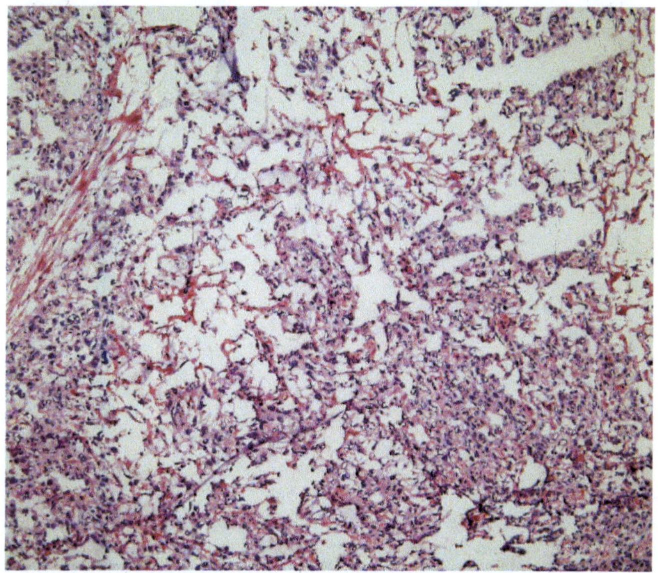

FIGURE 5.1 *Endodermal sinus tumor.* Microcystic and reticular patterns of an endodermal sinus tumor are seen in FS of a biopsy of a testicular mass in the planning for partial orchiectomy. However, the diagnosis of endodermal sinus tumor as revealed by FS requires radical orchiectomy. This is partly due to the fact that intratubular germ cell tumor is frequent in the adjacent testicular tissue.

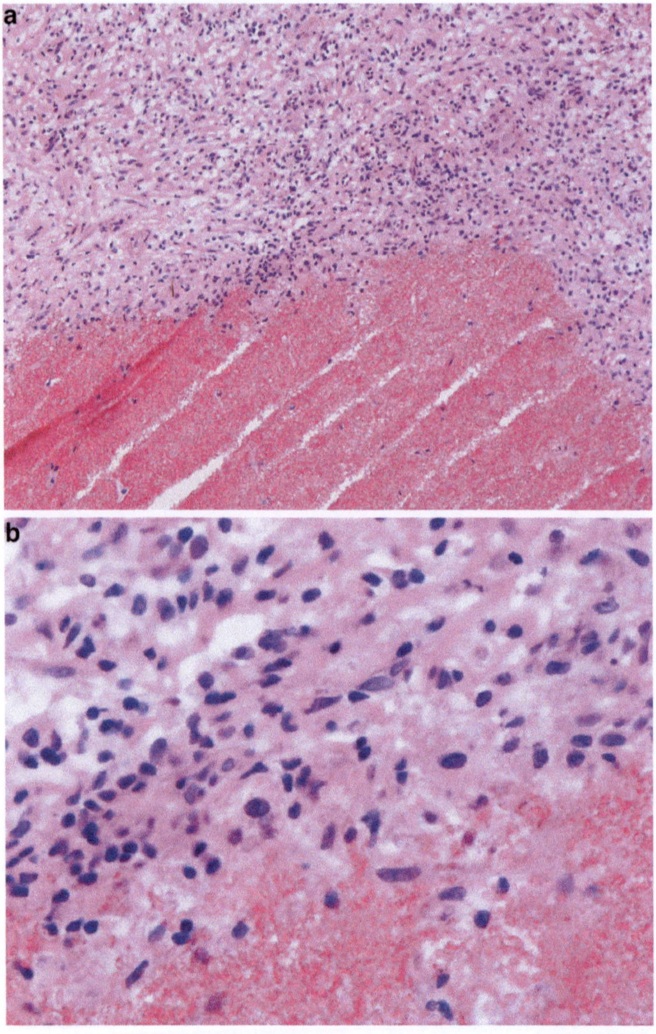

FIGURE 5.2 *Organizing hematoma.* (**a**) FS of a biopsy of a painful testicular mass in a 35-year-old man, showing a hematoma surrounded by fibrous tissue. (**b**) The tissue adjacent to the hematoma is composed of fibroblasts and small and large lymphoid cells, indicating a reactive process. Germ cell tumor can show extensive hemorrhagic necrosis, which must be differentiated from hematoma. The absence of necrosis, necrotic tumor cells, or viable tumor cells after careful sampling favors hematoma. A trauma was not recalled by the patient. No additional surgery was performed.

chiefly due to the high frequency of intratubular germ cell neoplasia in the remaining testicular tissue.[118,119]

Asymptomatic nonpalpable testicular lesions are being incidentally recognized with increasing frequency. Although they can be germ cell tumors that require radical orchiectomy, some of them might be benign tumors or non-neoplastic lesions that can be successfully treated by partial orchiectomy. FS consultation may be requested in this context for a definitive diagnosis. These lesions may include (1) Tumors in prepubertal patients, about 60% of which are benign.[120,121] However, about 13% of adult testicular tumors are benign, and these tumors may also benefit from testis-sparing surgery; (2) Nonpalpable testicular tumors detected by ultrasonography performed because of infertility, pain, or other symptoms; most of which are benign (Figs. 5.2 and 5.3);[122] and (3) Lesions, usually inflammatory or vascular in nature, which may mimic tumor, but may still be nonneoplastic by clinical or imaging findings (Fig. 5.4).

As mentioned above, partial orchiectomy is not indicated for germ cell tumor. However, it should be considered in the treatment of synchronous bilateral germ cell tumors or unilateral germ cell tumor with a history of contralateral orchiectomy for germ cell tumor (1–5% of cases). Under these circumstances, rather than FS consultation, testis-sparing surgery should be followed by biopsies of the surrounding parenchyma for permanent sections. If an intratubular germ cell tumor is present, the testis may be irradiated, in which case fertility will be lost, but not potency.[123]

Specimen Handling

There is no consensus on the way testis specimens for FS should be obtained and handled.

The specimen may represent biopsies of the lesion and it should be entirely submitted for FS. Although hemorrhagic or necrotic areas should be avoided by the urologist, this type of tissue may represent a major component of the biopsy. These areas may also harbor microscopic foci of high-grade germ cell tumor components, such as embryonal carcinoma or choriocarcinoma, justifying the recommendation that the entire submitted specimen, regardless of its gross appearance, should be submitted for FS.

If the tumor is small (<2 cm), the entire tumor with 2–5 mm grossly uninvolved parenchyma may be excised and submitted for intraoperative consultation.[124] The entire surgical margin should be inked, followed by serial sectioning to identify the lesion and its relation to the surgical margins. Both lesional and surgical margin tissues should be submitted, taking in consideration of the gross

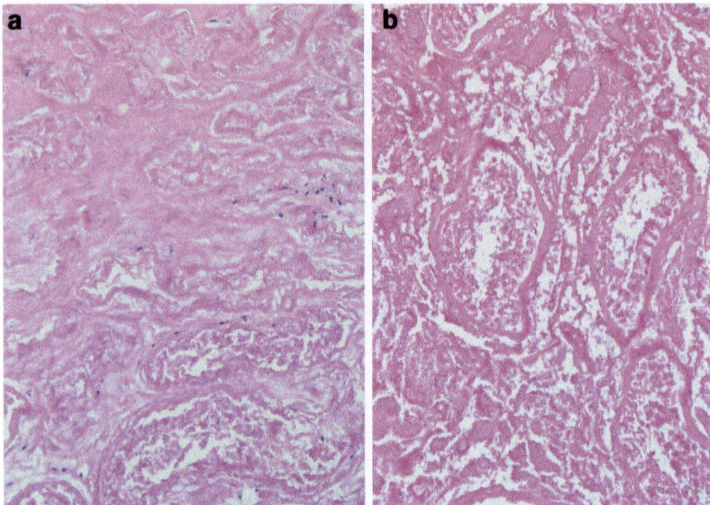

FIGURE 5.3 *Testicular infarct*. (**a**) On FS, the outer portion of the lesion is composed of virtually acellular hyalinized stroma and seminiferous tubule remnants. (**b**) The deeper portion of the lesion shows necrotic testicular tissue with intact architecture.

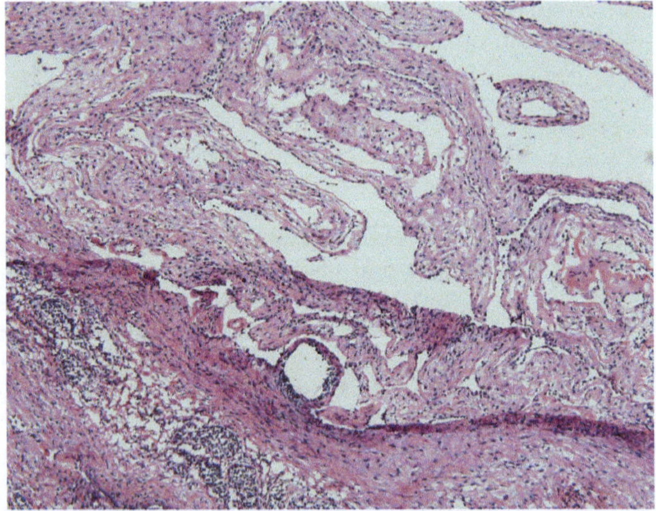

FIGURE 5.4 *Benign vascular tumor*. For partial orchiectomy, a lesion was sent for FS evaluation. There are only dialted lymphatic channels with no tumor or granuloma, justifying testis-sparing surgery.

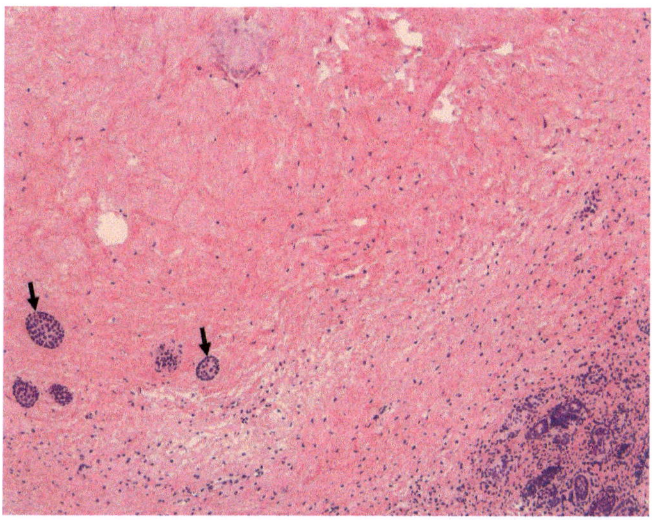

FIGURE 5.5 *Fibrous scar-like tissue.* This testicular lesion is thought to be benign and was excised by partial orchiectomy and submitted for FS, which demonstrates a dense collagenous scar-like tissue with no tumor. The arrows indicate residual seminiferrous tubules with Sertoli cells only. "Burnt-out" germ cell tumor is one of the differential diagnoses. However, the absence of intratubular germ cell tumor, as noted in this case, tends to negate this possibility.

appearance and the tumor size. Usually two sections are submitted for FS. In some cases, touch-imprint cytology can be useful.[125]

Random biopsy of the remaining testicular tissue is usually performed after partial orchiectomy (Figs. 5.5 and 5.6) to allow evaluation of the residual testicular tissue including the possibility of intratubular germ cell tumor. It is better to evaluate these biopsies on permanent sections, rather than FS.

If the FS is not definitive and the surgeon does not plan to excise the whole tumor before a definitive diagnosis is obtained, additional biopsies of the lesion and biopsies of the grossly uninvolved areas should be submitted for permanent sections.[126]

Interpretation

The diagnosis of the lesions includes benign (including determination of histological subtype if possible), malignant (including subtype if possible), or inconclusive lesion.[127] Distinguishing between benign and malignant lesions by FS is highly accurate (94.2–100%

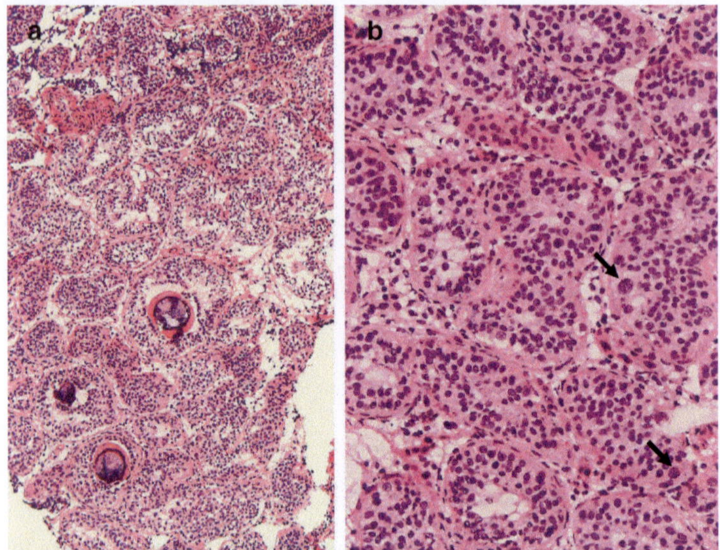

FIGURE 5.6 *Intratubular germ cell tumor (ITGCN)*. Submission of testicular tissue for FS diagnosis of ITGCN is usually not indicated. However, this type of FS may rarely occur since the identification of ITGCN may facilitate the diagnosis of germ cell tumor as implied in the case described in Fig 5.5. The FS diagnosis of ITGCN is problematic and is often deferred until permanent sections are obtained with ancillary immunostain. (**a**) Intratubular calcification may be associated with ITGCN, but a definitive diagnosis requires diagnostic tumor cells. (**b**) Seminiferrous tubules populated by a quite uniform population of cells, some of which are atypical (*arrows*). These findings are suspicious but not diagnostic for ITGCN.

being correct), but an inconclusive diagnosis is noted in about 13.3% of cases.[127]

Distinction between neoplasms is based on the cell types and growth patterns, which is often affected by FS artifacts. Thus, there are interpretation caveats in the context of FS, among which the following areas are highlighted:

Homogeneous clear cell pattern: Seminoma is typically composed of clear cells, and the tumor cells display characteristic nuclear features (Fig. 5.7). However, in FS, tumor cells may resemble foamy histiocytes, which together with the interstitial lymphocyte infiltrates frequently observed in seminoma can be mistaken for inflammatory lesions (nonspecific, xanthogranulomatous, or Rosai-Dorfman disease).[128,129] For the same considerations,

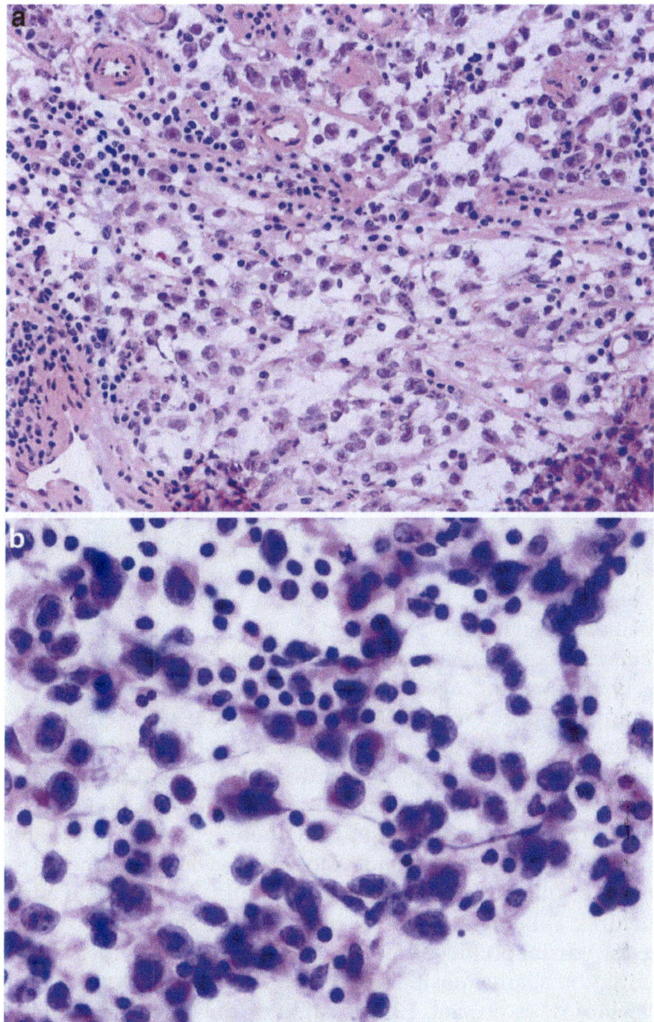

FIGURE 5.7 *Seminoma*. (**a**) FS shows typical cytologic features of tumor cells: abundant but flimsy cytoplasm, large pleomorphic nuclei, and prominent nucleoli. The characteristic lymphoid cell infiltration is also noted. (**b**) These features (seminomatous cells and lymphocytes) are also obvious in a touch preparation.

inflammatory processes may also be interpreted as seminoma with a marked inflammatory reaction. Another testicular clear cell neoplasm that poses a differential diagnosis with the seminoma that shows a tubular growth pattern (tubular seminoma) is Sertoli cell tumor.[130] The features that favor the diagnosis of Sertoli cell tumor include lack of mitosis, presence of nucleoli, and interstitial lymphocytic infiltrate, all of which are commonly seen in seminoma.

Granulomatous/lymphocytic components (Figs. 5.8–5.10): These are typically and frequently seen in seminoma. However, they rarely become so abundant to mask neoplastic cells, thus mimicking nonspecific chronic or granulomatous orchitis.[131] When the lymphocytic infiltrate is abundant, the differential diagnoses should include chronic orchitis, seminoma associated with a marked lymphocytic reaction, malignant lymphoma, and other lymphoproliferative processes.[132] Observations that can assist in differential diagnosis are the presence of seminoma cells, either scattered or clustered; the presence of multinucleated giant cells; the status of the seminiferous tubules trapped within the lesional areas (either preserved or infiltrated by lymphocytes); and the presence of atypical intratubular germ cells in the surrounding testicular parenchyma.

Teratomatous components (Figs. 5.11 and 5.12): The teratomatous component of a germ cell tumor has metastatic potential in postpubertal testes regardless of maturity, but it is benign in prepubertal testes.[133] While this component displays subtle morphological differences between these two age groups, it is the patient's age that is most helpful (usually less than 10 years of age for prepubertal teratoma and almost always between 20 and 40 years for postpubertal teratoma). Epidermoid cyst, which composed only of mature squamous epithelium and keratin, without skin adnexal structures, is benign regardless of the patient's age, and is a candidate for partial orchiectomy. A correct FS diagnosis including differentiation against postpubertal teratoma (which requires radical orchiectomy) is crucial. Examination of the entire specimen and the adjacent tissue for intratubular germ cell neoplasia and other skin adnexal structures (which should be absent in epidermoid cyst) is recommended.[134,135]

Differential diagnoses of germ cell tumor subtypes: It is often unnecessary to make a definitive diagnosis of the histological subtype of germ cell tumors intraoperatively, since their treatment is the same. Furthermore, although seminoma, the most frequent type of germ cell tumor, can be diagnosed in FS most of the times, its morphological spectrum is broad and some variants may mimic the other types of germ cell tumor.[136]

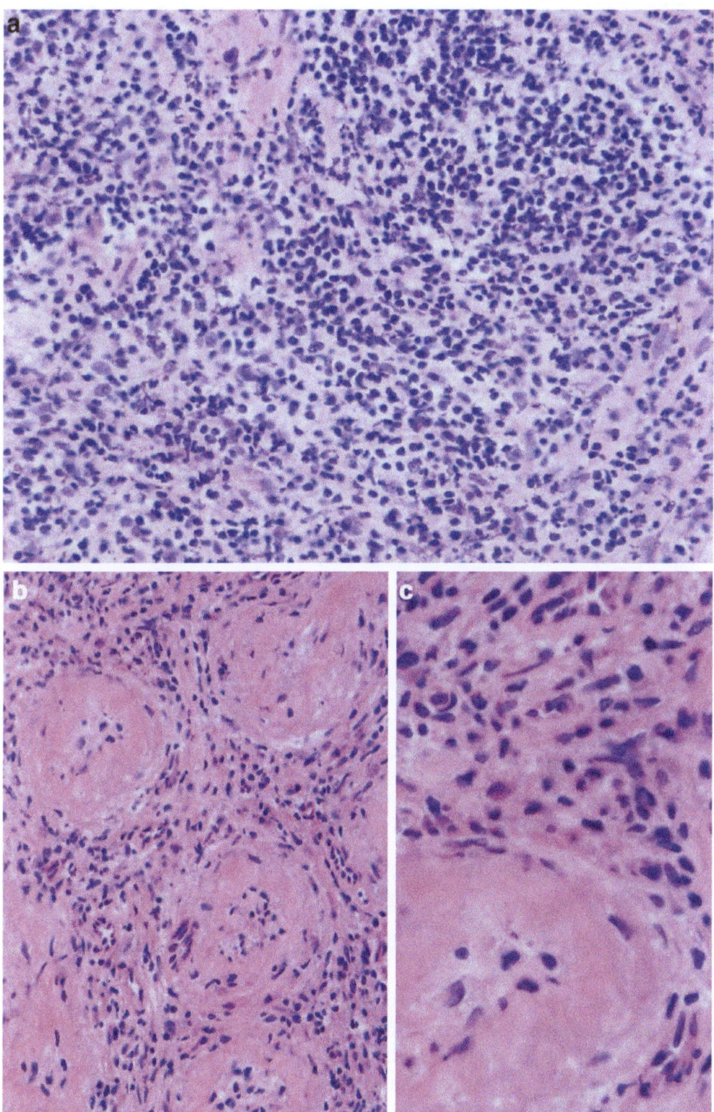

FIGURE 5.8 *Chronic orchitis*. (**a**) FS of a biopsy of a localized testicular mass in a 20-year-old man shows aggregation of small lymphoid cells. The differential diagnoses include chronic inflammation, seminoma, and lymphoma. (**b**, **c**): More biopsies were requested and they showed sclerotic seminiferous tubules separated by scattered small lymphoid cells, plasma cells, and benign spindle cells (probably fibroblasts). These features support the diagnosis of chronic orchitis. No additional surgery was performed.

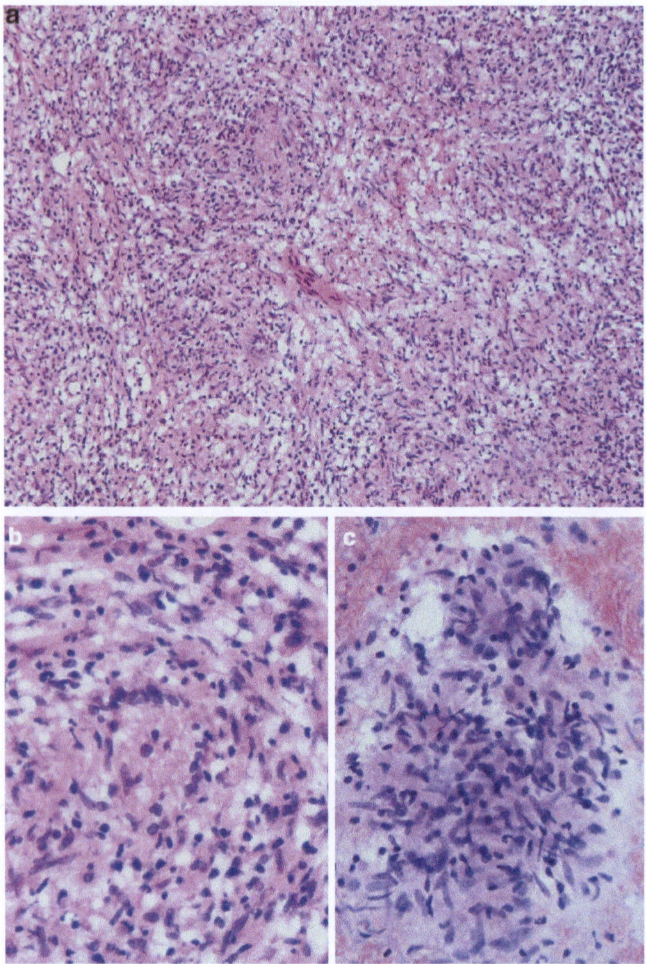

FIGURE 5.9 *Idiopathic granulomatous orchitis*. (**a**) FS of a biopsy of an ill-defined testicular lesion in a 57-year-old man showed nonnecrotizing granulomatous inflammation with a hint of ductulocentric distribution, without recognizable residual seminiferous tubules. Among the different causes of granulomatous orchitis, this pattern suggests the possibility of idiopathic granulomatous orchitis, rather than infectious or sarcoid etiology, in which the granulomatous inflammation tends to be interstitial and may show necrosis. (**b**) A granuloma with a multinucleated giant cell is noted. (**c**) Nonnecrotizing granulomas are sampled by touch preparation. Additional biopsy was requested for culture (which later showed no organisms). Because of the FS diagnosis, no additional surgery was performed. Idiopathic granulomatous orchitis is the most frequent mimicker of germ cell tumors.

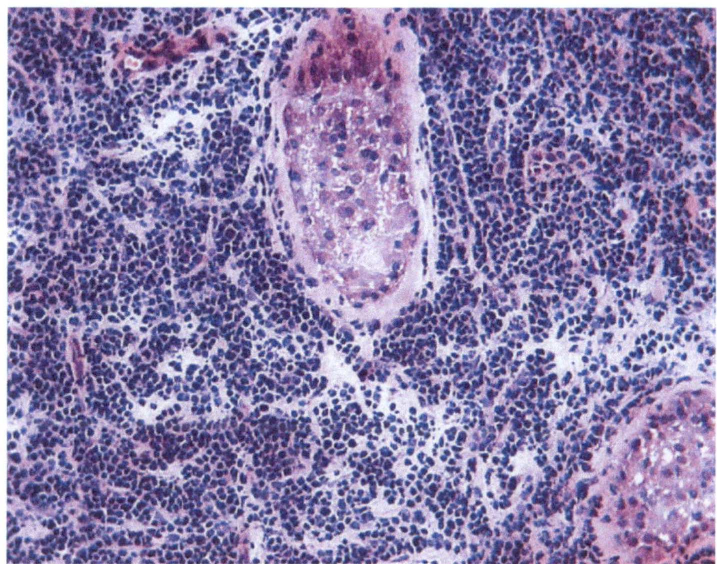

FIGURE 5.10 *Lymphoma*. Radical orchiectomy in a 65-year-old man. The interstitium is expanded by monotonous lymphoid cells. In such a case, even when FS is not requested, it may be performed at the discretion of the pathologist since a diagnosis of possible lymphoma calls for submission of fresh tissue for flow cytometry.

Nongerm cell tumors: Among these tumors, the stromal tumors are the most frequent including Leydig and Sertoli cell tumors. The solid growth of uniform cells without nuclear atypia, with eosinophilic cytoplasm, and the absence of interstitial lymphocytes facilitate the diagnosis of Leydig cell tumor.[137,138] Some authors report good results even with the touch imprints and scrape smear thanks to the presence of cytoplasmic Reinke crystalloids, typical for this tumor type.[139]

Sertoli cell tumor also can be identified by FS.[140] This type of tumor, however, is more difficult to distinguish from other neoplasms since its clear cell cytoplasm and variable growth patterns may be shared by other testicular tumors. Rare sex cord stromal tumors include granulosa cell tumor, mixed and unclassified sex cord stromal cell tumors.

The majority of these stromal tumors are benign. The malignant cases can exceptionally occur but it may not possible to identify them by morphological features alone.

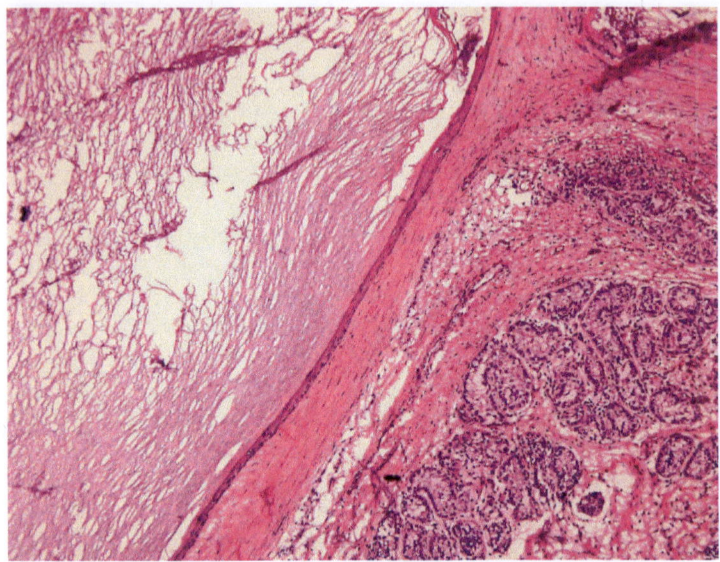

FIGURE 5.11 *Epidermoid cyst.* An incidental testicular mass in a boy is excised by partial orchiectomy. *Multiple* samples submitted to FS show that it is composed only of a mature squamous epithelial lining and keratinous material in the cystic lumen. Adjacent uninvolved testicular parenchyma of prepubertal appearance is seen. No additional surgery was needed.

Other benign tumors as adenomatoid tumor (Fig. 5.13)[141] or cystic dysplasia of the rete testis, especially in children,[142] must be considered in the differential diagnosis by FS. The vacuolated cytoplasm and the microscopic appearance of the cystic spaces and location of the lesions can help in the diagnosis.

Metastatic Tumors: Metastatic tumors rarely appear as a primary testicular mass at presentation (except in the case of malignant lymphoma), particularly in older age group. In patients with a clinical history of neoplasm elsewhere, any unusual morphology should raise the suspicion of a metastatic tumor. Distinction of these tumors from Sertoli cell tumor or neoplasia of paratesticular structures (rete testis, mesothelium, and epididymis) may be very difficult morphologically. In contrast, germ cell tumor can rarely mimic a metastatic carcinoma morphologically.[143] These situations have not been studied from the point of view of intraoperative pathological diagnosis, but it is obvious that the pathologist should report any unexpected aspect of the FS to the urologist, and both should then agree on the appropriate nature of the surgical intervention.

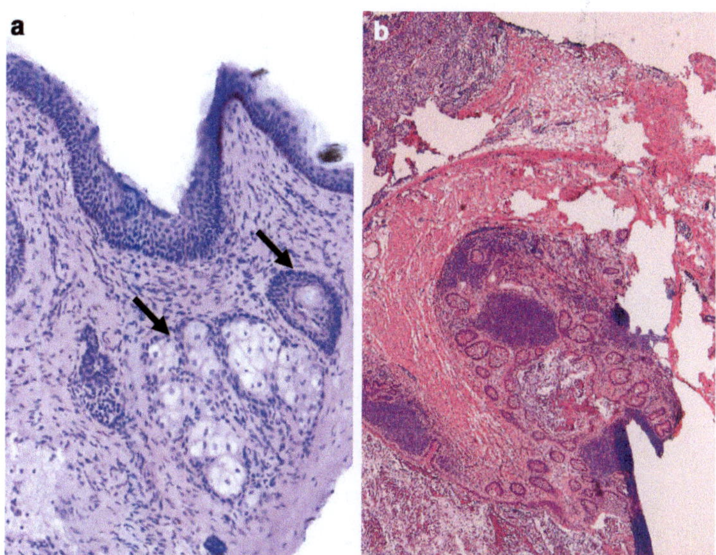

FIGURE 5.12 *Mature cystic teratoma*. (**a**) A small palpable testicular mass in a 10-year-old boy was removed by partial orchiectomy. FS of a portion of the tumor shows cystic spaces lined by mature squamous epithelium. Skin appendages (*arrows*) are also noted, raising the possibility of a mature cystic teratoma (which requires radical orchiectomy) rather than epidermoid cyst. (**b**) Additional tumor tissue sampling shows mature gastrointestinal wall and lymphoid tissue, diagnostic for mature cystic teratoma. Radical orchiectomy was then performed.

GROSS CONSULTATION/FROZEN SECTION OF LYMPH NODES IN RETROPERITONEAL NODAL DISSECTION

Clinical Background

The indications for retroperitoneal lymph node dissection in the treatment of germ cell tumor are variable. It may be performed for accurate staging for a nonseminomatous germ cell tumor without clinical nodal metastasis, before planning adjuvant chemotherapy. In nonseminomatous germ cell tumor with clinical evidence of nodal metastasis, the metastasis is usually treated with neoadjuvant chemotherapy, followed by retroperitoneal lymph node dissection if there is still residual tumor mass even when the serum markers normalize. The disadvantage of the radical lymphadenectomy is a loss of potency in 40–90% of patients. The risk of limited lymphadenectomy is tumor relapse. Because of these reasons and

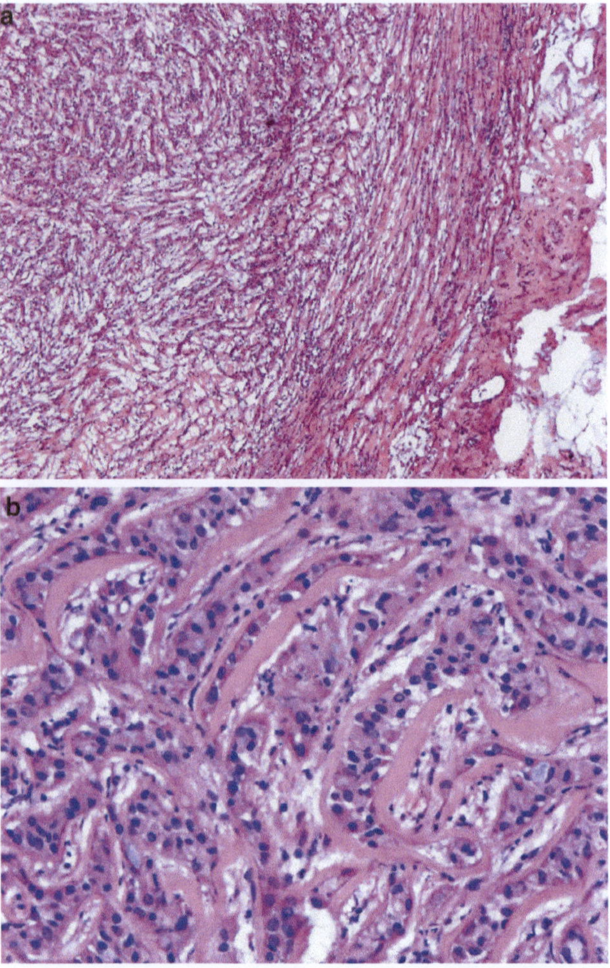

FIGURE 5.13 *Adenomatoid tumor*. (**a**) A 1.2 cm incidental "scrotal mass" in a 26-year-old man was excised with a thin rim of surrounding testicular tissue. The tumor is composed of cords and islands of tumor cells separated by edematous stroma. FS also shows that the tumor abuts the surgical margin, but in view of a benign tumor, the urologist elected to preserve testicular tissue, rather than additional excision. (**b**) Elongated cords of benign tumor cells surrounded by thickened basement membrane. Although adenomatoid tumor may display several different growth patterns, creating potential confusion with other tumors in testis or paratesticular organs, the features shown here are diagnostic for adenomatoid tumor, which permits testis-sparing surgery.

the observation that nodal spread of germ cell tumor is orderly (without "skipping" lesion), the surgeon may submit some lymph nodes for gross or FS consultation in order to determine the extent of retroperitoneal lymphadenectomy.

Specimen Handling

Frequently only gross consultation is needed. If multiple nodes are submitted, the biggest or grossly suspicious one should be submitted to FS. Rapid immunohistochemistry as an adjunct to FS has been reported but is not practical or helpful.[144]

Interpretation

FS report should first indicate whether metastatic tumor is present. If it is present, the type and the relative amount of the germ cell tumor components should be reported as well. If the lymph node is abnormal, but the grossly abnormal areas are totally necrotic or fibrotic without viable tumor component on FS, the findings should be reported to surgeon as a provisional diagnosis and the final result should be deferred until permanent sections, which may reveal focal viable tumor cells. The metastatic tumor may rarely show sarcomatous or carcinomatous transformation, which portends a poor prognosis.

FROZEN SECTION/TOUCH PREPARATION OF TESTICULAR BIOPSY IN THE CONTEXT OF MANAGEMENT OF INFERTILITY

Clinical Background

Absence of spermatozoa in the semen (azoospermia) is present in 10–15% of infertile men. It may be due to intrinsic pathological changes of the testicular tissue or obstruction of the semen outflow tract but with normal spermatogenesis. Differentiation between these conditions, which is possible by testicular biopsy and its touch preparation, is obviously important since microsurgical correction of the obstruction is often successful. Microsurgery may be attempted *after* the biopsy results, or *during* testicular biopsy. In the latter situation, intraoperative consultation is requested.[145-147]

Since only 20–40% of couples conceived after microsurgery in spite of a patent rate of 60–80%, there is recent attempt to obtain sperms from testis or from various locations in the semen outflow tract during the operation, and save them by cryopreservation for possible future in vitro fertilization. The same consideration is true for vasectomy reversal. The role of intraoperative consultation in this context is evolving.[147]

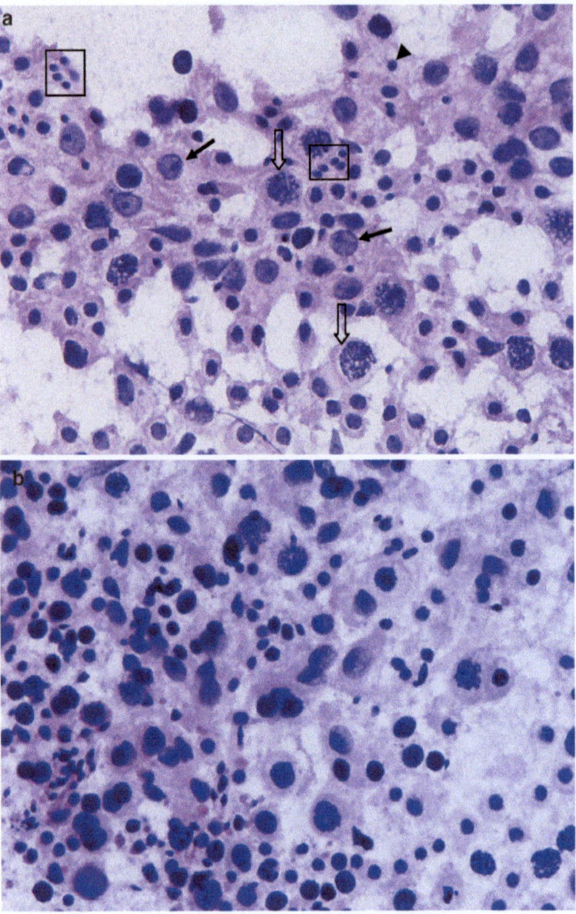

FIGURE 5.14 *Normal spermatogenesis*. (**a**) A well-prepared touch preparation displays Sertoli cells with abundant cytoplasm, open chromatin, and large nucleoli (*solid arrows*); primary spermatocytes with a characteristic chromatin pattern (*open arrows*); and several spermatozoa (*box*). Although not clearly visible in this picture, fine details of the spermatozoan including their tails can be appreciated in touch preparation. Other germ cells such as spermatids can also be seen (*arrow head*). The smear is characteristically cellular. (**b**) These fine details are lost in another smear from the same biopsy that is overstained. Germ cells are particularly susceptible to this type of artifact. This intraoperative touch preparation in the course of surgical management for azoospermia suggests an obstructive cause, allowing for immediate microsurgery to proceed.

Specimen Handling

One or more testicular biopsies by open or transcutaneous approach are submitted. Before submitting each of them for FS, touch preparation should be made. Touch preparation is essential since it allows the recognition of different testicular cell types including fine details such as the tail of spermatozoa, which may be difficult in even the best FS.[145] Since the biopsy is often small, there is temptation to touch the biopsy on the glass slide several times before fixation. This practice is discouraged since drying artifacts seem to develop more quickly and cause more morphological distortion in testicular tissue than for other tissue types. This consideration is also true for FS preparation. Although a rapid Romanowsky stain (diffQuik) has been proposed, it does not offer any advantage over the routine H&E stain.

Interpretation

The biopsy/touch preparation findings are complementary and may show one of four following patterns: normal spermatogenesis, hypospermatogenesis, maturational arrest, and "Sertoli cell-only"/germinal aplasia (Figs. 5.14–5.17). However, perhaps the only finding that needs to report is whether there are numerous morphologically normal spermatozoa, which suggests the possibility of obstructive azoospermia, potentially amenable to immediate microsurgical correction.[145]

EXAMINATION OF THE VASAL FLUID DURING VASECTOMY REVERSAL

Clinical Background

Vasectomy reversal may be achieved by different surgical procedures including vasovasostomy and vasoepididymyostomy. The choice of the surgical procedure, as well as the chance of successful restoration of fertility, may depend on the quality of the vasal fluid, which is obtained during the procedure and may be submitted for intraoperative consultation.[148]

Specimen Handling

The submitted vasal fluid should be put on a regular glass slide, coverslipped, and examined for spermatozoa. If the submitted vasal fluid has a thick creamy consistency, it should be diluted with normal saline before examination. After the diagnosis is rendered, the coverslip is removed and the slide is fixed in alcohol for routine H&E staining for permanent examination.[148]

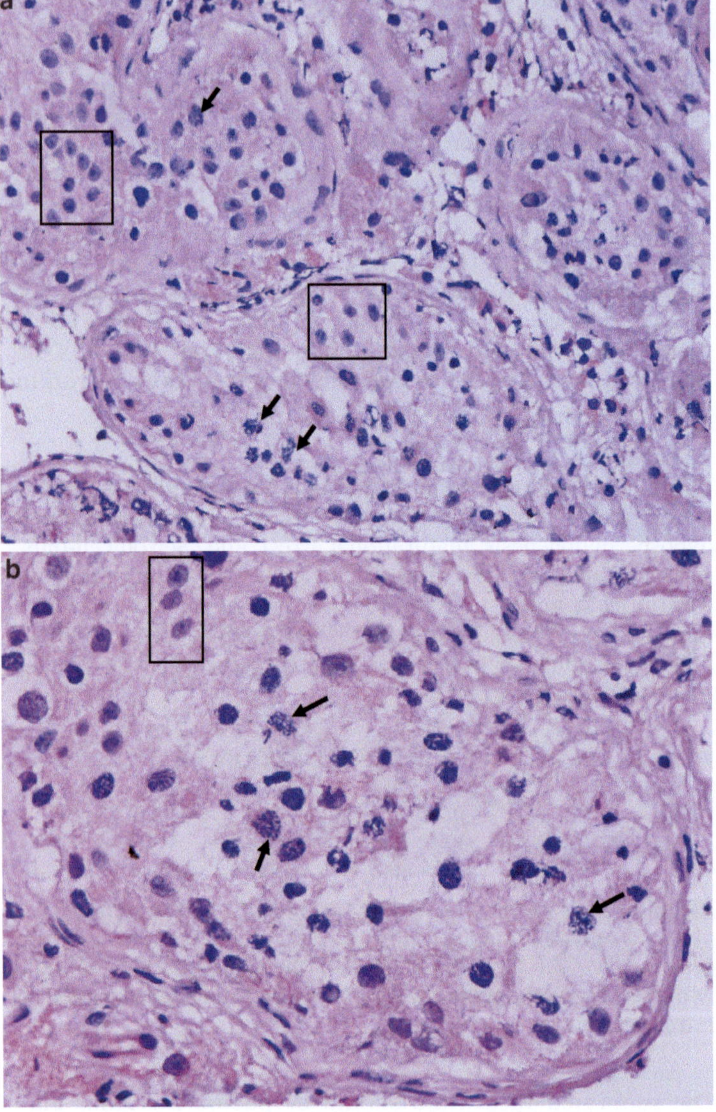

FIGURE 5.15 *Maturational arrest.* (**a**) FS of a testicular biopsy of a 36-year-old man with azoospermia shows that the seminiferous tubules are populated mostly by Sertoli cells (*boxes*). Primary spermatocytes (*arrows*) are also seen; other types of germ cells of undetermined nature (perhaps due to FS artifact) are also present. However, there are no spermatozoa. (**b**) High power view for better cytologic details.

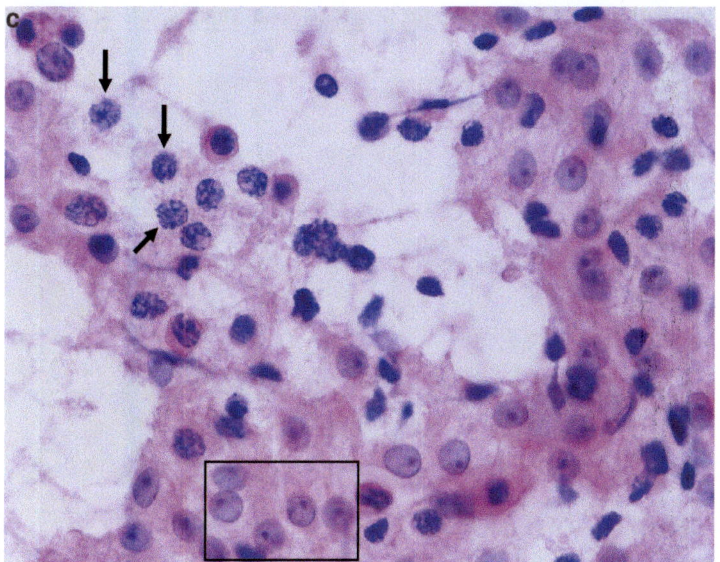

FIGURE 5.15 (continued) (**c**) The corresponding touch preparation shows the same cell types.

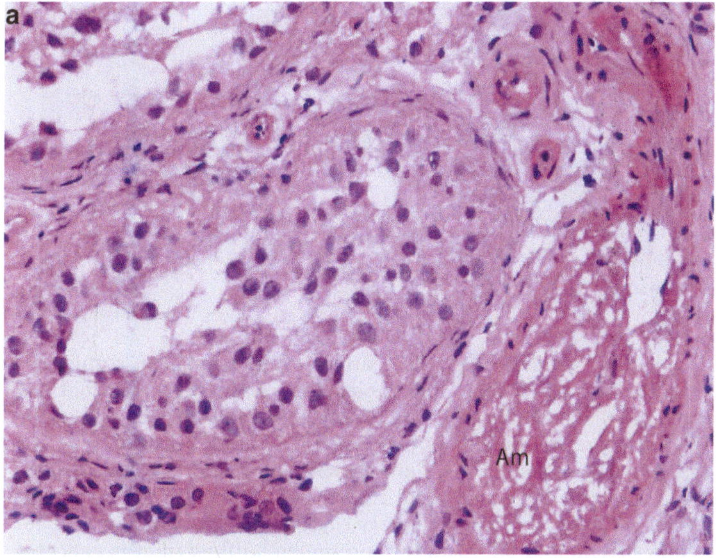

FIGURE 5.16 *"Sertoli cell only"*. (**a**) FS of the left testicular biopsy in a 31-year-old man with azoospermia shows a seminiferous tubule populated virtually by Sertoli cells only. Incidental prominent arterial wall eosinophilic deposition is noted (*Am*), the nature of which is not obvious on FS.

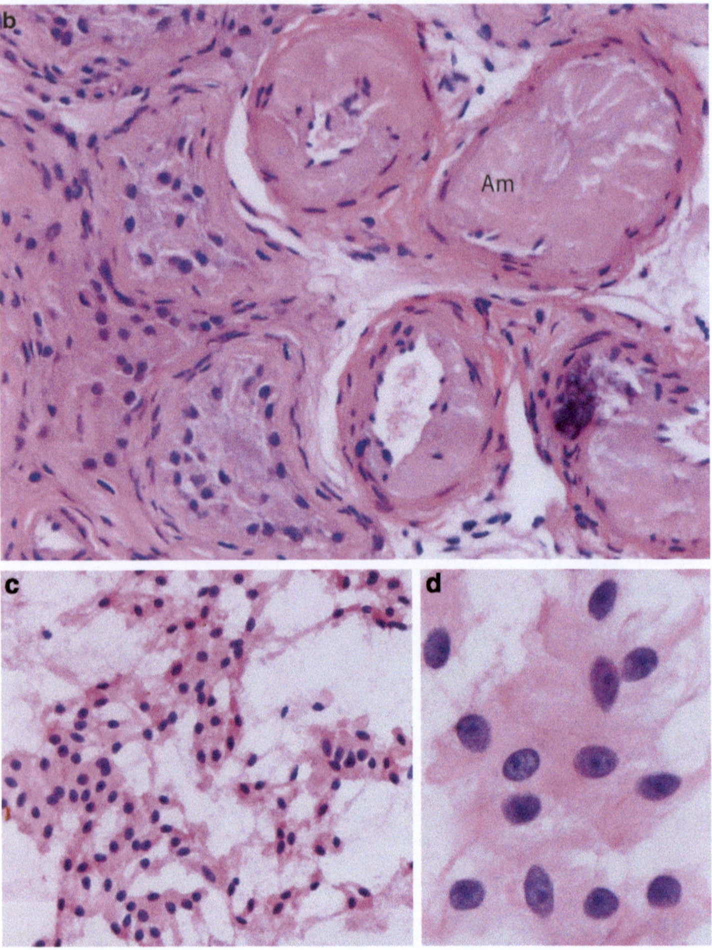

FIGURE 5.16 (continued) (**b**) The corresponding permanent section confirms the "Sertoli cell only" morphology and demonstrates amyloid (*Am*) in the vascular wall. The right testicular biopsy shows similar changes. (**c**): The touch preparation shows only abundant Sertoli cells, forming loose clusters. (**d**) The Sertoli cells show characteristic features including abundant cytoplasm, round or ovoid nuclei, fine chromatin, and prominent nucleoli. The intraoperative findings suggest that azoospermia is of testicular origin, and microsurgery on semen outflow tract is cancelled.

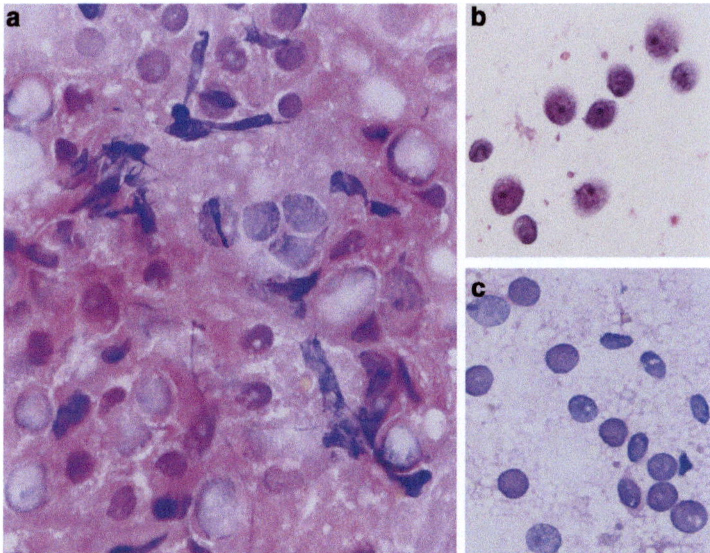

FIGURE 5.17 *"Sertoli cell only"* (**a**) Drying artifact in a smear prepared from the same biopsy as in Fig. 5.16 results in a marked loss of cellular details. (**b**) The cytoplasm of Sertoli cells is flimsy and can be lost during touch preparation, with preservation of nuclear details. (**c**) Cells with drying artifact and cytoplasmic loss. They are probably Sertoli cells but cannot be definitively identified as such.

5.6.3 Interpretation

The finding may be categorized as: Grade 1 = mainly normal motile spermatozoa, Grade 2 = mainly normal nonmotile spermatozoa, Grade 3: mainly sperm heads, Grade 4 = only sperm heads, and Grade 5 = no sperm. These findings may help with the surgical approach. For example, the 2008 practice guideline from the American Society of Reproductive Medicine suggests that vasovasostomy is performed for Grade 1–4 cases, whereas for Grade 5 cases, the choice between vasovasostomy and vasoepididymyostomy depends on other intraoperative findings.[148]

References

CHAPTER 1. KIDNEY

1. Oneson RH, Minke JA, Silverberg SG. Intraoperative pathologic consultation. An audit of 1,000 recent consecutive cases. Am J Surg Pathol. 1989;13:237–243.
2. Miller DC, Shah RB, Bruhn A, Madison R, Saigal CS. Trends in the use of gross and frozen section pathological consultations during partial or radical nephrectomy for renal cell carcinoma. J Urol. 2008;179:461–467.
3. Krishnan B, Lechago J, Ayala G, Truong L. Intraoperative consultation for renal lesions. Implications and diagnostic pitfalls in 324 cases. Am J Clin Pathol. 2003;120:528–535.
4. Blute ML, Leibovich BC, Cheville JC, Lohse CM, Zincke H. A protocol for performing extended lymph node dissection using primary tumor pathological features for patients treated with radical nephrectomy for clear cell renal cell carcinoma. J Urol. 2004;172:465–469.
5. Campbell SC, Fichtner J, Novick AC, et al. Intraoperative evaluation of renal cell carcinoma: a prospective study of the role of ultrasonography and histopathological frozen sections. J Urol. 1996;155:1191–1195.
6. Eble JN, Sauter S, Epstein JI, Sesterhenn IA. Pathology & Genetics of Tumors of the Urinary System and Male Genital Organs. Lyon: IARC Press; 2004.
7. Parsons MA, Harris SC, Longstaff AJ, Grainger RG. Xanthogranulomatous pyelonephritis: a pathological, clinical and aetiological analysis of 87 cases. Diagn Histopathol. 1983;6:203–219.
8. Dobyan DC, Truong LD, Eknoyan G. Renal malacoplakia reappraised. Am J Kidney Dis. 1993;22:243–252.
9. Silva EG, Kraemer B. Intraoperative Pathologic Diagnosis: Frozen Sections and Other Technique.: Wilkins & Williams; 1987.
10. Iskandar SS, Prahlow JA, White WL. Lipid-laden foamy macrophages in renal cell carcinoma. Potential frozen section diagnostic pitfall. Pathol Res Pract. 1993;189:549–552.

11. Amin MB, Crotty TB, Tickoo SK, Farrow GM. Renal oncocytoma: a reappraisal of morphologic features with clinicopathologic findings in 80 cases. Am J Surg Pathol. 1997;21:1–12.
12. Cochand-Priollet B, Molinie V, Bougaran J, et al. Renal chromophobe cell carcinoma and oncocytoma. A comparative morphologic, histochemical, and immunohistochemical study of 124 cases. Arch Pathol Lab Med. 1997;121:1081–1086.
13. Latham B, Dickersin GR, Oliva E. Subtypes of chromophobe cell renal carcinoma: an ultrastructural and histochemical study of 13 cases. Am J Surg Pathol. 1999;23:530–535.
14. Yip SK, Tan PH, Cheng WS, Li MK, Foo KT. Surgical management of angiomyolipoma: nephron-sparing surgery for symptomatic tumour. Scand J Urol Nephrol. 2000;34:32–35.
15. Uzzo RG, Novick AC. Nephron sparing surgery for renal tumors: indications, techniques and outcomes. J Urol. 2001;166:6–18.
16. Gill IS, Kavoussi LR, Lane BR, et al. Comparison of 1,800 laparoscopic and open partial nephrectomies for single renal tumors. J Urol. 2007;178:41–46.
17. Kubinski DJ, Clark PE, Assimos DG, Hall MC. Utility of frozen section analysis of resection margins during partial nephrectomy. Urology. 2004;64:31–34.
18. Breda A, Stepanian SV, Liao J, et al. Positive margins in laparoscopic partial nephrectomy in 855 cases: a multi-institutional survey from the United States and Europe. J Urol. 2007;178:47–50.
19. Eble JN. Angiomyolipoma of kidney. Semin Diagn Pathol. 1998;15:21–40.
20. de Peralta-Venturina M, Moch H, Amin M, et al. Sarcomatoid differentiation in renal cell carcinoma: a study of 101 cases. Am J Surg Pathol. 2001;25:275–284.
21. Grignon DJ, Eble JN. Papillary and metanephric adenomas of the kidney. Semin Diagn Pathol. 1998;15:41–53.
22. Ro JY, Ayala AG, el-Naggar A, Grignon DJ, Hogan SF, Howard DR. Angiomyolipoma of kidney with lymph node involvement. DNA flow cytometric analysis. Arch Pathol Lab Med. 1990;114:65–67.
23. Perez-Montiel D, Wakely PE, Hes O, Michal M, Suster S. High-grade urothelial carcinoma of the renal pelvis: clinicopathologic study of 108 cases with emphasis on unusual morphologic variants. Mod Pathol. 2006;19:494–503.
24. Kennedy SM, Merino MJ, Linehan WM, Roberts JR, Robertson CN, Neumann RD. Collecting duct carcinoma of the kidney. Hum Pathol. 1990;21:449–456.
25. Davis CJ, Jr., Mostofi FK, Sesterhenn IA. Renal medullary carcinoma. The seventh sickle cell nephropathy. Am J Surg Pathol. 1995;19:1–11.
26. Moncino MD, Friedman HS, Kurtzberg J, Pizzo SV. Papillary adenocarcinoma of the renal pelvis in a child: case report and brief review of the literature. Med Pediatr Oncol. 1990;18:81–86.
27. Warren KS, McFarlane JP. The Bosniak classification of renal cystic masses. BJU Int. 2005;95:939–942.
28. Todd TD, Dhurandhar B, Mody D, Ramzy I, Truong LD. Fine-needle aspiration of cystic lesions of the kidney. Morphologic spectrum and diagnostic problems in 41 cases. Am J Clin Pathol. 1999;111:317–328.

29. Truong LD, Krishnan B, Cao JT, Barrios R, Suki WN. Renal neoplasm in acquired cystic kidney disease. Am J Kidney Dis. 1995;26:1–12.

30. Watson ML. Complications of polycystic kidney disease. Kidney Int. 1997;51:353–365.

31. Eble JN, Bonsib SM. Extensively cystic renal neoplasms: cystic nephroma, cystic partially differentiated nephroblastoma, multilocular cystic renal cell carcinoma, and cystic hamartoma of renal pelvis. Semin Diagn Pathol. 1998;15:2–20.

32. Andonian S, Janetschek G, Lee BR. Laparoscopic partial nephrectomy: an update on contemporary issues. Urol Clin North Am. 2008;35:385–396.

33. Yossepowitch O, Thompson RH, Leibovich BC, et al. Positive surgical margins at partial nephrectomy: predictors and oncological outcomes. J Urol. 2008;179:2158–2163.

34. Lam JS, Bergman J, Breda A, Schulam PG. Importance of surgical margins in the management of renal cell carcinoma. Nat Clin Pract Urol. 2008;5:308–317.

35. Eroglu M, Unsal A, Bakirtas H, Tekdogan U, Ataoglu O, Balbay MD. Routine frozen-section biopsy from the surgical bed should be performed during nephron-sparing surgery for renal cell carcinoma. Scand J Urol Nephrol. 2005;39:222–225.

36. Lattouf JB, Beri A, D'Ambros OF, Grull M, Leeb K, Janetschek G. Laparoscopic partial nephrectomy for hilar tumors: technique and results. Eur Urol. 2008;54:409–416.

37. McHale T, Malkowicz SB, Tomaszewski JE, Genega EM. Potential pitfalls in the frozen section evaluation of parenchymal margins in nephron-sparing surgery. Am J Clin Pathol. 2002;118:903–910.

38. Li QL, Guan HW, Zhang QP, Zhang LZ, Wang FP, Liu YJ. Optimal margin in nephron-sparing surgery for renal cell carcinoma 4 cm or less. Eur Urol. 2003;44:448–451.

39. Tsuchiya K, Jinbo H, Kurita M, et al. Pathologic examination of renal cell cancer by means of step-sectioning. Int J Urol. 2000;7:335–339.

40. Baltaci S, Orhan D, Soyupek S, Beduk Y, Tulunay O, Gogus O. Influence of tumor stage, size, grade, vascular involvement, histological cell type and histological pattern on multifocality of renal cell carcinoma. J Urol. 2000;164:36–39.

41. Renshaw AA, Corless CL. Papillary renal cell carcinoma. Histology and immunohistochemistry. Am J Surg Pathol. 1995;19:842–849.

42. Tickoo SK, Reuter VE, Amin MB, et al. Renal oncocytosis: a morphologic study of fourteen cases. Am J Surg Pathol. 1999;23:1094–1101.

43. Bernie JE, Albers L, Baird S, Parsons CL. Synchronous ipsilateral renal adenocarcinoma, transitional cell carcinoma of the renal pelvis and metastatic renal lymphoma. J Urol. 2000;164:773–774.

44. Jimenez RE, Eble JN, Reuter VE, et al. Concurrent angiomyolipoma and renal cell neoplasia: a study of 36 cases. Mod Pathol. 2001;14:157–163.

45. Solomon D, Schwartz A. Renal pathology in von Hippel-Lindau disease. Hum Pathol. 1988;19:1072–1079.

46. Walther MM, Choyke PL, Glenn G, et al. Renal cancer in families with hereditary renal cancer: prospective analysis of a tumor size threshold for renal parenchymal sparing surgery. J Urol. 1999;161:1475–1479.

47. Steinbach F, Novick AC, Zincke H, et al. Treatment of renal cell carcinoma in von Hippel-Lindau disease: a multicenter study. J Urol. 1995;153:1812–1816.
48. Lubensky IA, Pack S, Ault D, et al. Multiple neuroendocrine tumors of the pancreas in von Hippel-Lindau disease patients: histopathological and molecular genetic analysis. Am J Pathol. 1998;153:223–231.
49. Truong LD, Caraway N, Ngo T, Laucirica R, Katz R, Ramzy I. Renal lymphoma. The diagnostic and therapeutic roles of fine-needle aspiration. Am J Clin Pathol. 2001;115:18–31.
50. Anderson CM, Pusztai L, Palmer JL, Cabanillas F, Ellerhorst JA. Coincident renal cell carcinoma and nonHodgkin's lymphoma: the M. D. Anderson experience and review of the literature. J Urol. 1998;159:714–717.
51. Pantuck AJ, Zisman A, Dorey F, et al. Renal cell carcinoma with retroperitoneal lymph nodes: role of lymph node dissection. J Urol. 2003;169:2076–2083.
52. Walker PD, Cavallo T, Bonsib SM. Practice guidelines for the renal biopsy. Mod Pathol. 2004;17:1555–1563.
53. Hefter LG, Brennan GG. Transillumination of renal biopsy specimens for rapid identification of glomeruli. Kidney Int. 1981;20:411–415.
54. Corwin HL, Schwartz MM, Lewis EJ. The importance of sample size in the interpretation of the renal biopsy. Am J Nephrol. 1988;8:85–89.
55. Colvin RB, Cohen AH, Saiontz C, et al. Evaluation of pathologic criteria for acute renal allograft rejection: reproducibility, sensitivity, and clinical correlation. J Am Soc Nephrol. 1997;8:1930–1941.
56. Racusen LC, Solez K, Colvin RB, et al. The Banff 97 working classification of renal allograft pathology. Kidney Int. 1999;55:713–723.
57. Sung RS, Christensen LL, Leichtman AB, et al. Determinants of discard of expanded criteria donor kidneys: impact of biopsy and machine perfusion. Am J Transplant. 2008;8:783–792.
58. Randhawa P. Role of donor kidney biopsies in renal transplantation. Transplantation. 2001;71:1361–1365.
59. Munivenkatappa RB, Schweitzer EJ, Papadimitriou JC, et al. The Maryland aggregate pathology index: a deceased donor kidney biopsy scoring system for predicting graft failure. Am J Transplant. 2008;8:2316–2324.
60. Gaber LW, Moore LW, Alloway RR, Amiri MH, Vera SR, Gaber AO. Glomerulosclerosis as a determinant of posttransplant function of older donor renal allografts. Transplantation. 1995;60:334–339.
61. Pastural M, Barrou B, Delcourt A, Bitker MO, Ourahma S, Richard F. Successful kidney transplantation using organs from a donor with disseminated intravascular coagulation and impaired renal function: case report and review of the literature. Nephrol Dial Transplant. 2001;16:412–415.
62. Colvin RB, Nickeleit V. Renal transplant pathology. In: Jennette JC, Olson JL, Schwartz MM, Silva FG, eds. Heptinstall's Pathology of the Kidney. 6th ed.: Lippincott Williams & Wilkins; 2007:1347–1490.

63. Wunderlich H, Wilhelm S, Reichelt O, Zermann DH, Borner R, Schubert J. Renal cell carcinoma in renal graft recipients and donors: incidence and consequence. Urol Int. 2001;67:24–27.
64. Ditonno P, Lucarelli G, Bettocchi C, et al. Incidentally discovered yellowish lesions in a renal graft from a deceased donor. Transplant Proc. 2008;40:2062–2064.
65. Penn I. Primary kidney tumors before and after renal transplantation. Transplantation. 1995;59:480–485.

CHAPTER 2.   URINARY BLADDER

66. Whitehair JG, Griffey SM, Olander HJ, Vasseur PB, Naydan D. The accuracy of intraoperative diagnoses based on examination of frozen sections. A prospective comparison with paraffin-embedded sections. Vet Surg. 1993;22:255–259.
67. Gephardt GN, Zarbo RJ. Interinstitutional comparison of frozen section consultations. A college of American Pathologists Q-Probes study of 90,538 cases in 461 institutions. Arch Pathol Lab Med. 1996;120:804–809.
68. Schoenberg MP, Walsh PC, Breazeale DR, Marshall FF, Mostwin JL, Brendler CB. Local recurrence and survival following nerve sparing radical cystoprostatectomy for bladder cancer: 10-year followup. J Urol. 1996;155:490–494.
69. Schumacher MC, Scholz M, Weise ES, Fleischmann A, Thalmann GN, Studer UE. Is there an indication for frozen section examination of the ureteral margins during cystectomy for transitional cell carcinoma of the bladder? J Urol. 2006;176:2409–2413.
70. Raj GV, Tal R, Vickers A, et al. Significance of intraoperative ureteral evaluation at radical cystectomy for urothelial cancer. Cancer. 2006;107:2167–2172.
71. Silver DA, Stroumbakis N, Russo P, Fair WR, Herr HW. Ureteral carcinoma in situ at radical cystectomy: does the margin matter? J Urol. 1997;158:768–771.
72. Stein JP, Clark P, Miranda G, Cai J, Groshen S, Skinner DG. Urethral tumor recurrence following cystectomy and urinary diversion: clinical and pathological characteristics in 768 male patients. J Urol. 2005;173:1163–1168.
73. Ashley RA, Inman BA, Sebo TJ, et al. Urachal carcinoma: clinicopathologic features and long-term outcomes of an aggressive malignancy. Cancer. 2006;107:712–720.
74. Ugurlu O, Adsan O, Tul M, Kosan M, Inal G, Cetinkaya M. Value of frozen sections of lymph nodes in pelvic lymphadenectomy in patients with invasive bladder tumor. Int J Urol. 2006;13:699–702.
75. Adsan O, Baltaci S, Cal C, et al. Reliability of frozen section examination of external iliac, hypogastric, and obturator lymph nodes during radical cystectomy: a multicenter study. Urology. 2007;69:83–86.

CHAPTER 3. PENIS

76. Hoffman MA, Renshaw AA, Loughlin KR. Squamous cell carcinoma of the penis and microscopic pathologic margins: how much margin is needed for local cure? Cancer. 1999;85:1565–1568.
77. Zhu Y, Ye DW, Chen ZW, Zhang SL, Qin XJ. Frozen section-guided wide local excision in the treatment of penoscrotal extramammary Paget's disease. BJU Int. 2007;100:1282–1287.
78. Ornellas AA, Seixas AL, de Moraes JR. Analyses of 200 lymphadenectomies in patients with penile carcinoma. J Urol. 1991;146:330–332.
79. Abi-Aad AS, deKernion JB. Controversies in ilioinguinal lymphadenectomy for cancer of the penis. Urol Clin North Am. 1992;19:319–324.

CHAPTER 4. PROSTATE

80. Fromont G, Baumert H, Cathelineau X, Rozet F, Validire P, Vallancien G. Intraoperative frozen section analysis during nerve sparing laparoscopic radical prostatectomy: feasibility study. J Urol. 2003;170:1843–1846.
81. Fasolis G, Degiuli P, Lancia M, et al. Periprostatic tissues intraoperative frozen section during retrograde radical retropubic prostatectomy. Arch Ital Urol Androl. 2006;78:107–111.
82. Goharderakhshan RZ, Sudilovsky D, Carroll LA, Grossfeld GD, Marn R, Carroll PR. Utility of intraoperative frozen section analysis of surgical margins in region of neurovascular bundles at radical prostatectomy. Urology. 2002;59:709–714.
83. Dillenburg W, Poulakis V, Witzsch U, et al. Laparoscopic radical prostatectomy: the value of intraoperative frozen sections. Eur Urol. 2005;48:614–621.
84. Kausik SJ, Blute ML, Sebo TJ, et al. Prognostic significance of positive surgical margins in patients with extraprostatic carcinoma after radical prostatectomy. Cancer. 2002;95:1215–1219.
85. Shah O, Melamed J, Lepor H. Analysis of apical soft tissue margins during radical retropubic prostatectomy. J Urol. 2001;165:1943–1948.
86. Lepor H, Kaci L. Role of intraoperative biopsies during radical retropubic prostatectomy. Urology. 2004;63:499–502.
87. Nazeer T, Kee KH, Ro JY, et al. Intraprostatic adipose tissue: a study of 427 whole mount radical prostatectomy specimens. Hum Pathol. 2009;40:538–541.
88. Ayala AG, Ro JY, Babaian R, Troncoso P, Grignon DJ. The prostatic capsule: does it exist? Its importance in the staging and treatment of prostatic carcinoma. Am J Surg Pathol. 1989;13:21–27.
89. Billis A. Intraprostatic fat: does it exist? Hum Pathol. 2004;35:525.
90. Chuang AY, Epstein JI. Positive surgical margins in areas of capsular incision in otherwise organ-confined disease at radical prostatectomy: histologic features and pitfalls. Am J Surg Pathol. 2008;32:1201–1206.

91. Partin AW, Kattan MW, Subong EN, et al. Combination of prostate-specific antigen, clinical stage, and Gleason score to predict pathological stage of localized prostate cancer. A multi-institutional update. JAMA. 1997;277:1445–1451.

92. Kakehi Y, Kamoto T, Okuno H, Terai A, Terachi T, Ogawa O. Peroperative frozen section examination of pelvic nodes is unnecessary for the majority of clinically localized prostate cancers in the prostate-specific antigen era. Int J Urol. 2000;7:281–286.

93. Beissner RS, Stricker JB, Speights VO, Coffield KS, Spiekerman AM, Riggs M. Frozen section diagnosis of metastatic prostate adenocarcinoma in pelvic lymphadenectomy compared with nomogram prediction of metastasis. Urology. 2002;59:721–725.

94. Epstein JI. Pathologic assessment of the surgical specimen. Urol Clin North Am. 2001;28:567–594.

95. Epstein JI, Oesterling JE, Eggleston JC, Walsh PC. Frozen section detection of lymph node metastases in prostatic carcinoma: accuracy in grossly uninvolved pelvic lymphadenectomy specimens. J Urol. 1986;136:1234–1237.

96. Davis GL. Sensitivity of frozen section examination of pelvic lymph nodes for metastatic prostate carcinoma. Cancer. 1995;76:661–668.

97. Schned AR, Gormley EA. Florid xanthomatous pelvic lymph node reaction to metastatic prostatic adenocarcinoma. A sequela of preoperative androgen deprivation therapy. Arch Pathol Lab Med. 1996;120:96–100.

98. Wilcox GE, Conway EJ, Wheeler TM, Truong LD. Benign glandular inclusions detected in pelvic lymph nodes removed during staging of prostate adenocarcinoma. Mod Pathol. 1998;11:99A.

99. Gazdar AF. Tumors arising after organ transplantation. Sorting out their origins. JAMA. 1997;277:154–155.

100. Mikuz G, Montironi R, Lopez-Beltran A, Bussolati G. The dilemma of multiorgan donors with high serum PSA – a pathologist"s proposal. Virchows Arch. 2006;449:273–276.

101. Algaba F, Arce Y, Lopez-Beltran A, Montironi R, Mikuz G, Bono AV. Intraoperative frozen section diagnosis in urological oncology. Eur Urol. 2005;47:129–136.

102. Geddy PM, Reid IN. Selective sampling of yellow prostate chips: a specific method for detecting prostatic adenocarcinoma. Urol Int. 1996;56:33–35.

103. Algaba F, Epstein JI, Aldape HC, et al. Assessment of prostate carcinoma in core needle biopsy – definition of minimal criteria for the diagnosis of cancer in biopsy material. Cancer. 1996;78:376–381.

104. Ro JY, Amin MB, Kim KR, Ayala AG. Tumors and tumorous conditions of the the male genital tract. In: Fletcher, CDM, ed. Diagnostic Histopathology of Tumors. 3rd ed.. London: Churchill Livingstone; 2007:749–879.

105. Molinie V, Fromont G, Sibony M, et al. Diagnostic utility of a p63/alpha-methyl-CoA-racemase (p504s) cocktail in atypical foci in the prostate. Mod Pathol. 2004;17:1180–1190.

106. Helpap B. Small suggestive lesions of the prostate. Histological and immunohistochemical analyses – report of the uropathology consultation service. Pathologe. 2005;26:398–404.
107. Bonkhoff H, Remberger K. Benign microglandular prostate lesions. Diagnostic criteria na differential diagnosis. Pathologe. 1998;19:1–11.
108. Algaba F, Trias I. Diagnostic limits in precursor lesions of prostatic cancer. Eur Urol. 1996;30:212–221.
109. Srigley JR. Benign mimickers of prostatic adenocarcinoma. Mod Pathol. 2004;17:328–348.
110. Grignon DJ, Ro JY, Srigley JR, Troncoso P, Raymond AK, Ayala AG. Sclerosing adenosis of the prostate gland. A lesion showing myoepithelial differentiation. Am J Surg Pathol. 1992;16:383–391.
111. Bostwick DG, Chang L. Overdiagnosis of prostatic adenocarcinoma. Semin Urol Oncol. 1999;17:199–205.
112. Epstein JI, Walsh PC, Sanfilippo F. Clinical and cost impact of second-opinion pathology. Review of prostate biopsies prior to radical prostatectomy. Am J Surg Pathol. 1996;20:851–857.
113. Thorson P, Swanson PE, Vollmer RT, Humphrey PA. Basal cell hyperplasia in the peripheral zone of the prostate. Mod Pathol. 2003;16:598–606.
114. Kaleem Z, Swanson PE, Vollmer RT, Humphrey PA. Prostatic adenocarcinoma with atrophic features: a study of 202 consecutive completely embedded radical prostatectomy specimens. Am J Clin Pathol. 1998;109:695–703.
115. Di Silverio F, Monti S, Sciarra A, et al. Effects of long-term treatment with Serenoa repens (Permixon) on the concentrations and regional distribution of androgens and epidermal growth factor in benign prostatic hyperplasia. Prostate. 1998;37:77–83.
116. Malpica A, Ro JY, Troncoso P, Ordonez NG, Amin MB, Ayala AG. Nephrogenic adenoma of the prostatic urethra involving the prostate gland: a clinicopathologic and immunohistochemical study of eight cases. Hum Pathol. 1994;25:390–395.
117. Rahemtullah A, Oliva E. Nephrogenic adenoma: an update on an innocuous but troublesome entity. Adv Anat Pathol. 2006;13:247–255.

CHAPTER 5. TESTIS

118. Bahrami A, Ro JY, Ayala AG. An overview of testicular germ cell tumors. Arch Pathol Lab Med. 2007;131:1267–1280.
119. van Casteren NJ, Boellaard WP, Dohle GR, et al. Heterogeneous distribution of ITGCNU in an adult testis: consequences for biopsy-based diagnosis. Int J Surg Pathol. 2008;16:21–24.
120. Dodat H, Chavrier Y, Dyon JF, et al. Primary testicular tumors in children. Apropos of 23 cases. Chirurgie pediatrique. 1986;27:1–13.
121. Lin JN, Wang KL, Chuang JH. Primary testicular tumors in children. Int Surg. 1988;73:190–192.

122. Sheynkin YR, Sukkarieh T, Lipke M, Cohen HL, Schulsinger DA. Management of nonpalpable testicular tumors. Urology. 2004;63:1163–1167.

123. Hughes PD. Partial orchidectomy for malignancy with consideration of carcinoma in situ. ANZ J Surg. 2006;76:92–94.

124. Hopps CV, Goldstein M. Ultrasound guided needle localization and microsurgical exploration for incidental nonpalpable testicular tumors. J Urol. 2002;168:1084–1087.

125. Hoda RS, Hoda SA, Reuter VE. Intraoperative touch-imprint cytology of germ cell neoplasms. Diag Cytopathol. 1996;14:393–394.

126. Elert A, Olbert P, Hegele A, Barth P, Hofmann R, Heidenreich A. Accuracy of frozen section examination of testicular tumors of uncertain origin. Eur Urol. 2002;41:290–293.

127. Leroy X, Rigot JM, Aubert S, Ballereau C, Gosselin B. Value of frozen section examination for the management of nonpalpable incidental testicular tumors. Eur Urol. 2003;44:458–460.

128. Fernandopulle SM, Hwang JS, Kuick CH, et al. Rosai-Dorfman disease of the testis: an unusual entity that mimics testicular malignancy. J Clin Pathol. 2006;59:325–327.

129. Al-Said S, Ali A, Alobaidy AK, Mojeeb E, Al-Naimi A, Shokeir AA. Xanthogranulomatous orchitis: review of the published work and report of one case. Int J Urol. 2007;14:452–454.

130. Young RH. Testicular tumors – some new and a few perennial problems. Arch Pathol Lab Med. 2008;132:548–564.

131. Pickard WR, Clark AH, Abel BJ. Florid granulomatous reaction in a seminoma. Postgrad Med J. 1983;59:334–335.

132. Mehta HH, Thirumala S, Palestro CJ. Leukemic infiltration mimicking epididymo-orchitis on scrotal scintigraphy. Clin Nucl Med. 1997;22:721–722.

133. Mostert M, Rosenberg C, Stoop H, et al. Comparative genomic and in situ hybridization of germ cell tumors of the infantile testis. Lab Invest. 2000;80:1055–1064.

134. Wiesenthal JD, Ettler H, Razvi H. Testicular epidermoid cyst: a case report and review of the clinicopathologic features. Can J Urol. 2004;11:2133–2135.

135. Maizlin ZV, Belenky A, Baniel J, Gottlieb P, Sandbank J, Strauss S. Epidermoid cyst and teratoma of the testis: sonographic and histologic similarities. J Ultrasound Med. 2005;24:1403–1409.

136. Ulbright TM, Young RH. Seminoma with tubular, microcystic, and related patterns: a study of 28 cases of unusual morphologic variants that often cause confusion with yolk sac tumor. Am J Surg Pathol. 2005;29:500–505.

137. Carmignani L, Colombo R, Gadda F, et al. Conservative surgical therapy for Leydig cell tumor. J Urol. 2007;178:507–511.

138. Giannarini G, Mogorovich A, Menchini Fabris F, et al. Long-term followup after elective testis sparing surgery for Leydig cell tumors: a single center experience. J Urol. 2007;178:872–876.

139. Hribar KP, Warner NE, Sherrod AE. Cytologic identification of Reinke crystalloids in scrapings and imprints of fresh testicular tumors: a simple and rapid technique for intraoperative use. Arch Pathol Lab Med. 2005;129:e65–e66.

140. Nagata M, Kurimoto S, Takeuchi T, Ohta N, Minowada S, Kitamura T. Tiny nodule in the testicle: case report of a Sertoli cell tumor. Int J Urol. 2004;11:61–62.

141. Medina Perez M, Sanchez Gonzalez M. [Paratesticular adenomatoid tumor, presentation as epididymal pain]. Arch Esp Urol. 1998;51:88–90.

142. Van Kote G, Leconte D, Renault D, Godefroy Y, Charbonnel E. [Benign cystic tumors of the testis in children]. Chir Pediatr. 1987;28:102–107.

143. Ulbright TM, Young RH. Metastatic carcinoma to the testis: a clinicopathologic analysis of 26 nonincidental cases with emphasis on deceptive features. Am J Surg Pathol. 2008;32:1683–1693.

144. Stosiek P, Wodke A, Kasper M. Immunohistological detection of lymph node metastases in the testicular center as quick section diagnosis during retroperitoneal lymphadenectomy. Pathol Res Pract. 1993;189:1010–1014.

145. Kim ED, Greer JA, Abrams J, Lipshultz LI. Testicular touch preparation cytology. J Urol. 1996;156:1412–1414.

146. Kim ED, Gilbaugh JH, 3rd, Patel VR, Turek PJ, Lipshultz LI. Testis biopsies frequently demonstrate sperm in men with azoospermia and significantly elevated follicle-stimulating hormone levels. J Urol. 1997;157:144–146.

147. The Practice Committee of the American Society for Reproductive Medicine. Evaluation of the azoospermic male. Fertil Steril. 2008;90 (5 Suppl):S74–S77.

148. The Practice Committee of the American Society for Reproductive Medicine. Vasectomy reversal. Fertil Steril. 2008;90 (5 Suppl):S78–S82.

Index

V

X

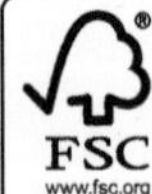

MIX
Papier aus verantwortungsvollen Quellen
Paper from responsible sources
FSC® C105338

If you have any concerns about our products,
you can contact us on
ProductSafety@springernature.com

In case Publisher is established outside the EU,
the EU authorized representative is:
Springer Nature Customer Service Center GmbH
Europaplatz 3, 69115 Heidelberg, Germany

Printed by Libri Plureos GmbH
in Hamburg, Germany